Computers in Health Care

Kathryn J. Hannah   Marion J. Ball
Series Editors

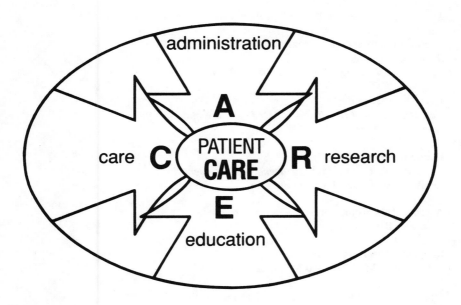

Computers in Health Care

Series Editors:
Kathryn J. Hannah   Marion J. Ball

Michael K. Bourke

Strategy and Architecture of Health Care Information Systems

With 143 Illustrations

Springer-Verlag
New York Berlin Heidelberg London Paris
Tokyo Hong Kong Barcelona Budapest

Michael K. Bourke, Ph.D.
Associate Professor of Information Systems
Director, MS in Management, Computing, and Systems
College of Business and Economics
Houston Baptist University
7502 Fondren Road
Houston, TX 77074-3298, USA

Library of Congress Cataloging-in-Publication Data
Bourke, Michael K.
Strategy and architecture of health care information systems / by
Michael K. Bourke.—1st ed.
    p.   cm.—(Computers and health care)
Includes bibliographical references and index.
ISBN 0-387-97982-4 (New York).—ISBN 3-540-97982-4 (Berlin)
1. Medical informatics.   2. Hospital records.   3. Information
storage and retrieval systems—Medicine.   I. Title.   II. Series.
R858.B675   1994
362.1'1'0285—dc20   93-27727

Printed on acid-free paper.

Production coordinated by Chernow Editorial Services, Inc., and managed by Natalie
Johnson; manufacturing supervised by Jacqui Ashri.
Typeset by Best-set Typesetter Ltd., Hong Kong.
Printed and bound by Edwards Brothers, Inc., Ann Arbor, MI.
Printed in the United States of America.

9 8 7 6 5 4 3 2 1

ISBN 0-387-97982-4 Springer-Verlag New York Berlin Heidelberg
ISBN 3-540-97982-4 Springer-Verlag Berlin Heidelberg New York

To Timothy and Alison

Series Preface

This series is intended for the rapidly increasing number of health care professionals who have rudimentary knowledge and experience in health care computing and are seeking opportunities to expand their horizons. It does not attempt to compete with the primers already on the market. Eminent international experts will edit, author, or contribute to each volume in order to provide comprehensive and current accounts of innovations and future trends in this quickly evolving field. Each book will be practical, easy to use, and well referenced.

Our aim is for the series to encompass all of the health professions by focusing on specific professions, such as nursing, in individual volumes. However, integrated computing systems are only one tool for improving communication among members of the health care team. Therefore, it is our hope that the series will stimulate professionals to explore additional means of fostering interdisciplinary exchange.

This series springs from a professional collaboration that has grown over the years into a highly valued personal friendship. Our joint values put people first. If the Computers in Health Care series lets us share those values by helping health care professionals to communicate their ideas for the benefit of patients, then our efforts will have succeeded.

Kathryn J. Hannah
Marion J. Ball

Acknowledgments

I owe thanks to the following people: Dr. Ralph Feigin, Physician-in-Chief of Texas Children's Hospital, who encouraged me to do the book when others said it could not be done; to Dr. Greg Buffone, John Espinosa, Linda Howell, Ron Wolfe, Holly Boyd, and Vicki Wiest, all from Texas Children's Hospital; and to Mike Hadley, from HBO & Company, Inc.

Contents

1
Introduction

Like many American industries, health care has undergone a fundamental restructuring in the past ten years, and it faces signficant change throughout the 1990s. Health care has gone from a relatively stable industry to a dynamic one. Even though most hospitals still look the same, the industry has changed fundamentally. The government has changed the way that it reimburses hospitals for Medicare/Medicaid patients. Consumer attitudes have changed. There is a nursing shortage. Payer practices have changed. Doctor behaviors have changed. Hospital attitudes towards patients have changed. Hospital attitudes towards management have changed. Many management disciplines, previously unknown or unneeded in hospital management, have been adopted by hospitals. They include marketing, product line management, cost accounting, materials management, and information systems architecture. Information systems management in hospitals has been particularly weak historically.

When the structure of an industry changes, the rules of competition change. This means that individual organizations have to change just to survive, to say nothing of prospering. Change requires rethinking one's position within the industry, and redesigning one's business processes (behaviors), which in turn also requires new information technology and new methods for its management. Like organizations, information systems have been designed to function within a particular industry model, and they have to be changed when the model changes.

When one examines information systems across numerous industries, one finds that the state of information systems in any organization reflects the state of that organization's general management. Most systems fail, not for technical reasons, but for reasons of general management: the wrong people made the decision, priorities were not set; projects were not controlled; behaviors were not changed; plans were not made, and so forth. In previous competitive environments, IS failures, while costly, were usually not fatal. However, in the changed environment, such failures could be disastrous. For that reason, general management needs to learn additional "survival" skills—approaches to information and technology management.

Vendors are advertising technology as a way to give hospitals a "competitive advantage." Unfortunately, the skill set possessed by general managers does not predispose them to attempt such decisions; hence this book. It is meant to provide an approach for thinking strategically about information systems: how they relate to the industry's changing structure, how they relate to the hospital's business processes, and how they relate to each other (systems integration). The concept of "fit" is at the heart of strategic thinking, and at the heart of this book. Does a strategy "fit" with the environment? Does it "fit" with the hospital's culture and structure? Does one hospital activity "fit" with another? Do information systems "fit" with the processes they are supposed to support?

In order for a "fit" to occur, the major stakeholders in IS decisions must have a shared conceptual understanding of the issues. In that spirit, the book is ambitious in defining its readership. It is intended for the following diverse segments: general hospital management (CEO, VPs, and department heads), hospital technical management, other hospital technical staff, vendors and consultants, and educators.

1. *General Hospital Management*: These individuals set strategies and make decisions, but they are removed from the business processes and the technology, so they avoid making decisions about these areas. As the paradigm for the hospital industry changes, the paradigm for hospital information systems structure also changes. As hospitals redesign their model for patient care, they will have to redesign their Information Systems (IS) model. However, in order to redesign IS, one has to change many other hospital processes that impact the effectiveness of IS. This includes strategy and planning, performance measurement, risk management, organizational design, reward systems, control systems, prioritization systems, and data management. These are all generic management activities, but they occur within the context of technology. Because of this, they are avoided, or done inappropriately. This book provides models for understanding the technical context. General management can read the whole book, hopefully even the technical sections of Chapters 4, 5, and 6. Each of these three chapters is divided into three sections: General, Management, and Technical. The general and management sections are designed to provide sufficient material for the general manager to feel comfortable in a technical context. If time allows, the general manager should be able to read the technical section. It has many details, but managers are now being required to know more and do more. The flattening of organizations is the result of companies discovering that layers of management do not do anything of value. They are too far from

the business process and too far from the strategy, and know nothing about technology.

2. *Technical Management*: This includes CIOs and VPs of information systems. Just as general management does not have a good way of discussing technical issues, so technical management does not have a good way of discussing strategy and business process. The book aims to provide them with insights into the linkages between systems strategy and business strategy, and between business processes and the systems that support them. It should allow them to present more effectively their requests for resources and standards. A large number of CIOs feel more comfortable discussing either business processes or technology, but not both. This book should help fill in the knowledge gaps.

3. *Other Technical Staff*: This includes both Hospital Information Systems (HIS) staff and end users who are involved in the systems development process. The book provides them with a big picture of the strategy and business processes. The more a developer understands about the background and context of the system, the more effective his design and analysis work, and his support of the users, will be. This group includes staff who go by the titles of Systems Analyst, Industrial Engineer, Management Engineer.

4. *Users*: Like general management, users of information systems may not want to take the time to read the technical sections of Chapters 4–6. Otherwise, they should be able to read the whole book. It should help them in defining their requirements, and in improving their business processes.

5. *Consultants and Vendors*: These individuals should gain some insights into the linkages between hospital information systems and organizations. The book should give consultants ideas on how to communicate with their clients during engagements, particularly on issues such as enterprise redesign/integration through technology. Vendors need to present their products as solutions to business problems. Heretofore, they have done a poor job of couching their systems in business terms. They do poorly in explaining how their solution fits the hospital's processes and existing systems architecture. They also have not done the best job of "architecting" their own systems. This audience includes other third parties such as payers, regulators, and suppliers, who want to gain insights into the health care industry and its information needs.

6. *Educators*: Graduate programs such as the MHA may also find this material useful. If one intends to teach hospital management, then management of the fit between systems and business processes is an important area to cover.

This book was not written just for large hospitals, even though they tend to have more complex systems and larger technical staffs than the smaller hospitals. In many ways, this book may prove more useful to the smaller hospital, by providing a conceptual framework for the use of consultants. Consultants and other third parties can provide the personnel to help overcome the resource surges and expertise shortfalls associated with systems development projects. However, consultants cannot be managed effectively if the hospital cannot frame the technical issues or define what it expects to get out of the engagement, or explain what the overall course of the engagement should look like. This book should be of value, whether a hospital develops its own systems from scratch or purchases them from a vendor. The basic issues remain: strategy and architecture, alignment of the business process, and controls.

Approach

The organizing principle of this book is an architectural metaphor, summarized in Figure 1.1. Any hospital is a collection of business processes. These business processes use data and are supported by technology. The business processes need to be organized effectively (Business Architecture); the data needs to be organized effectively (Data Architecture); and the technology needs to be organized effectively (Technical Architecture). Furthermore, there must be an alignment among these three elements. The degree of alignment is determined by the control systems of the hospital. These were mentioned previously; they include: strategy and planning, performance measurement, risk management, organizational design, reward systems, control systems, prioritization systems, and data management.

Every manager within an organization needs to know something about the other processes. The general manager needs to understand his business processes, as well as the data and technology that underlie them. The

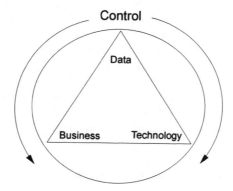

Figure 1.1 The architectures of a business.

technical manager needs to understand the business processes that he is supporting with technology. All parties need to understand how to design the many organizational structures and policies (controls) that assure the alignment among business process, data, and technology.

The book uses models to illustrate most points. The author's experience in consulting, management, education, and systems analysis has shown that the use of models is indispensable. They serve three functions: communication, analysis, and management of complexity. Using a model to illustrate a concept forces the proponent of the idea to articulate his thoughts more clearly; it also allows the audience to assimilate the concept more effectively, because the model presents something common and tangible about which both parties can agree. This is nothing new. Planners have models; financial analysts have models; accountants have models (the chart of accounts). The book is eclectic, using multiple models. It draws upon models of strategic planning, industrial engineering, data modeling, and general systems analysis and design techniques.

The book proceeds from strategy to architecture, from architecture to methodology, and from methodology to a mock strategic plan. While there is a consciously designed logical flow from one chapter to another, each can be read with relative independence. Chapter 1 provides an introduction. Chapter 2 provides an overview of the history of the health care industry in America. This sets the stage for discussion of the structural characteristics of health care, strategic issues, and models for strategy. Chapter 3 presents the history of health care information systems. This sets the stage for discussion of the linkages between systems and business strategy. Chapter 4 (Business Architecture) links business strategy with the processes that implement it. It presents models and methods for redesigning these business processes. Chapter 5 (Data Architecture) discusses the strategic importance of data. It also presents models and methods for aligning data with the business processes. Chapter 6 (Technical Architecture) discusses networking, and provides models and methods for aligning IS technology with the processes it supports. Chapter 7 (Control Architecture) examines the organizational design that is needed to ensure an effective linkage among strategy, process, data, and technology. Chapter 8 (Abbreviated Methodology) presents an outline of a methodology for developing a strategic plan and a systems architecture. Chapter 9 presents possible future developments and how they might impact strategy and health care systems architecture. Chapter 10 presents a mock IS Strategic Plan, which is intended to unify and make tangible many of the concepts discussed in the chapters on architecture.

It is both risky and frustrating to write a book that deals with technology, because technology becomes outdated very quickly. For this reason, trends are presented, rather than detailed solutions. The primary focus of this book is *methodology*, not technology, and so the book treats technology as an enabling device, not as an end in itself. Methodologies have a longer life cycle than technologies. Once strategy and architecture are understood, individual technologies can be used as they become available. This book also deals with standards, such as HL7 (for health care data exchange), which are evolving, but which will not be obsolete in the near future. For the same reason, the book avoids detailed discussion of the individual features of vendor systems. Vendors are continually upgrading their systems. Also, it is difficult to discuss any single feature out of context.

Other Sources

Some excellent books have been written on the subject of health care information systems. Richard Sneider (*Management Guide to Health Care Information Systems*, Aspen Publishers, 1987) contains a detailed survey of health care information systems vendors and applications. It gives a history of the different types of health care information systems and their technologies, and a guide to systems vendors. Joseph DeLuca (*Health Care Information Systems: An Executive's Guide for Successful Management*, American Hospital Publishing, 1991) presents an overview of management issues regarding systems planning, systems selection, systems installation, and systems management.

This book is intended to fill the niche left open by Sneider and DeLuca: how to set up the strategy and architecture against which vendor and system decisions must be made.

2
Health Care Industry Structure

Chapter 2 takes a structural look at the health care industry circa 1994 and also provides a brief summary of the major events and trends that have led to the current situation.

History of the Health Care Industry

The nature of the health care industry has changed over time, with shifts in the dynamic equilibrium formed by economic, political, social, and technological factors. There have been five distinct periods since World War II: 1945–1965, 1965–1973, 1973–1983, 1983–1991, and 1991 and beyond.[1]

Health Care 1945–1965

This period was marked by general economic expansion, caused by U.S. emergence from the war as a military and economic colossus. Medical care was drawn into this economic expansion and became a major industry. There was a low supply and high demand for health care. Much of this demand was stimulated by the U.S. government. It was building an infrastructure in many areas: roads, utilities, and hospitals. This era saw a major expansion of medical school power, with increased government investment in health care research (previously, most funding had been received from private sources—either charitable agencies or private com-

---

[1] For a comprehensive treatment of the subject, see Paul Starr, *The Social Transformation of American Medicine*, New York: Basic Books, 1982.

panies). In 1946, passage of the Hill-Burton Act stimulated hospital construction by providing federal funds for the building of hospitals, with little government control. At this time, raw materials for all U.S. industries were relatively cheap. *Hosp. Recieve Gov. money — in Return — Hosp must give X amt. of $'s in free care.*

Health Care 1965–1973

The year 1965 saw passage of legislation for Medicare (A and B) and Medicaid. Emphasis now shifted from expansion of health care facilities and services to their equitable distribution. In the early 1960s it was decided that the government could afford to make high-quality health care available to all citizens who were unable to pay for it themselves. This influx of newly insured patients continued to fuel the rapid expansion of health care facilities.

A parallel phenomenon was the use of health care benefits as a substitute for increased salary. Health care benefits were used more and more to attract and retain workers in many industries. Like the government programs, this created a situation where the direct consumer of health care bore little, if any, burden for its payment.

In some respects, health care became like a regulated utility. There were no limits placed on demand. What resulted was a sheltered industry, relatively free from competition. The organizational impacts on hospitals were: (1) relatively low levels of management skills—there is no pressure to manage when margins are assured; (2) little need to develop information systems—there was no need for feedback and control and decision-making; (3) small, relatively unsophisticated in-house data processing staffs. The latter is partly explained by the large number of small (less than 200 beds) hospitals.

Health Care 1973–1983

The year 1973 marked the end of an era for the United States. In that year, the U.S. let the dollar float against gold, an explicit admission that the dollar no longer had its previous purchasing power, having been undermined by inflation—the result of increased public spending on the Vietnam War and social programs without a commensurate increase in taxes or productivity. Nineteen seventy-three also signaled a period of disenchantment with the health care policies of the past. The validity of two assumptions now came into question: (1) the belief that Americans need more health care, to be provided by the government; and (2) the belief that health care professionals and the existing system of nonprofit hospitals were best qualified to determine how these services were to be provided. This judgment now shifted to the government. By 1974, legislation was passed requiring all states to have Certificate of Need programs.

Gov. Sponsored Health Care

Emphasis now shifted from equity of distribution to cost control. This did not help, however. Health care expenditures as a percentage of the national budget continued to increase faster than any other component. There arose a new feeling that private institutions and alternative delivery systems could do it more cost effectively. Investor-owned hospitals began to proliferate. More HMOs were founded; however, efforts to launch them on a national scale were not very successful.

H.C. Facilites were Not Cost effective

Health Care 1983–1991

The percentage of the population eligible for government-provided health care continued to increase. Health care costs continued to grow. DRG legislation was passed in 1983, by which the government placed a cap on what it would reimburse hospitals for the inpatient care they provided to Medicare citizens. This caused a temporary flattening of government cost growth, but did nothing for the other groups that pay for health care. At the same time, employer-subsidized health care benefits continued to be viewed by employees as an entitlement, and the costs for employers rose because demand for services had no checks placed on it. The government's price controls led to cost shifting. Hospitals raised their rates knowing that the government would not pay the full amount, but that insurers would. This caused large employers and insurers to adopt a more active role in cost containment, introducing copayments and increased deductibles into their policies. This, in turn, rippled over onto their employees, the direct consumers of care, who became more discriminating buyers of insurance. The number of alternate providers, such as HMOs and PPOs, grew.

DRGs had a traumatic effect on hospital managements. Almost overnight, the health care industry was forced to behave "competitively." It had to manage its costs—to try to make do with less. It had to secure its supply of patients. This also impacted hospitals' management of their patients, insurers, physicians, and in-house staff.

"Management" implies decision making, and decision making requires the appropriate data. This data, in many cases, must be captured and analyzed by some information system. The new types of data that were needed were obvious: cost data, staff productivity, patient data, patient clinical data (to satisfy the government regulators), price data, physician data, market data. Very few systems existed for this purpose.

Data Extremely Important

Saw M.R. as Part of Revenue to Hosp

Health Care 1991 and Beyond

Despite DRGs, health care costs continued to increase, reaching 13 percent of the Gross National Product in 1991 and 14 percent in 1992. Several significant events occurred in this time frame. The state of Minnesota went to outcomes-based reimbursement for its providers. The state of Oregon applied for a Medicaid waiver so that it could rank what treatments it would pay for. A national practitioner data base was set up. In most major cities large employers banded into consortiums to build data bases correlating cost, outcome, and satisfaction data for the hospitals in that city. FASB ruled that companies must place future health care expenditures for retirees as a liability on their balance sheets. Attention was drawn to the large number of "medically indigent"—those people who are employed, but do not earn enough to pay for health care. Every major stakeholder (AMA, AHA, AARP, politicians, and think tanks) submitted a plan for health care reform. This showed universal dissatisfaction with the general system. All this, combined with President Clinton's promise to make health care reform a priority, guarantees even more fundamental restructuring of the industry.

Structural Model

One way to assess the impact of all these changes on one's hospital is to examine them using Michael Porter's Five Factors Model.[1] The health care industry can be viewed as five interrelated components: the industry segment, its suppliers, its customers, potential new entrants into the segment, and substitutes. This is presented in Figure 2.1. The box in the middle of the diagram represents the industry segment and the traditional industry rivals that compete within this segment. Each company has its own strategy and structure—some are more effective than others. They interact with their suppliers and customers. Suppliers not only provide tangible inputs for products, they also provide human resources and capital; they can also provide regulation (e.g., the government). Customers can also be entities that have a stake in the success of the company. An organization's goal is to achieve "leverage" over its suppliers and customers (causing customers to buy at favorable prices and suppliers to sell at favorable prices), or to prevent them from achieving leverage over the company.

Leverage is a complex concept. Supplier leverage results from several things: their concentration, the quality of the item supplied, the availability of alternate suppliers, and the availability of substitute inputs. Likewise, customer leverage results from their concentration, the structure of the distribution channels, the number of segment rivals, and their perception of the quality of what one is selling.

The industry rivals gain leverage over their suppliers in many ways: (1) There are too many suppliers, (2) the item supplied is a commodity, (3)

---

[1] We will use the models elaborated by Michael Porter in *Competitive Advantage*, New York: Free Press, 1985.

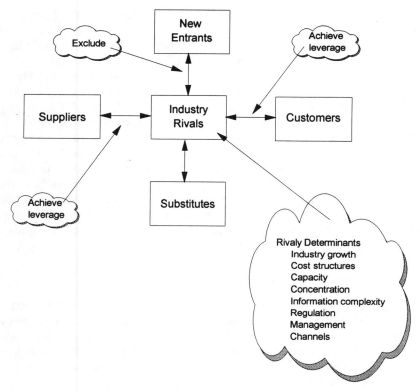

Figure 2.1 Five Factors model.

some event has occurred within the suppliers' industry that causes them to need cash quickly, (4) the rivals have economies of buying power, (5) physical location of suppliers. Leverage over suppliers translates into a lower cost of input goods and services. Conversely, if suppliers have leverage, they can charge higher prices.

The same holds true vis-à-vis customers. Higher leverage translates into higher prices. Conversely, customer leverage drives the price of the product down. The industry rivals gain leverage over them in similar ways: (1) Customer demand is not price sensitive, (2) demand is created through customer perception that the product has high value, (3) the customers are small and do not have economies of scale, (4) the customers do not have discretion over when they purchase the product, (5) there are few industry rivals supplying the product.

New entrants represent a threat to the traditional rivals. They threaten to drive prices down, drive costs up, take market share away from traditional rivals, or drive the traditional rivals out of the industry. Substitute products are alternatives to the products offered by the traditional industry.

In some industries, government and regulators play a stronger role than others. Health care is an example of this.

The underlying assumption is that leverage results in market share, which results in profitability. This has been corroborated through studies, which show that market share is disproportionately correlated to profitability. That is, if a company's market share grows, then its profitability will grow even more. But emphasis must be placed on the proper sequence of events: If you do things right, then your market share will grow, and thus your profits. Focusing on increasing profitability first does not ensure that market share will grow, and in the long run cannot produce the higher profits. Companies must understand the industry structure so that they can form strategies that will reshape the industry to their advantage. (It should be emphasized that if several rivals have the same strategy, then it is execution that will win.)

Health Care Industry Structure

The Five Factors model for the health care industry circa 1991–1992 is provided in Figure 2.2. The middle box represents the traditional rivals within the various health care industry segments: for-profit hospitals, not-for-profit hospitals, community and government hospitals, religious hospitals, and so forth. Their products are medical treatments of various kinds. They have different target populations for these medical services. These populations can be viewed by demographics (geriatric, pediatric, adult), by financial status (insured, self-pay, charity), by life-style, and other criteria.

The suppliers of goods and services are: real estate and construction, hospital supplies, medical equipment, information systems, insurance, and so forth. The customers (customer/payers) are: insurance companies, employers, government, patients, physicians, and other hospitals (when a patient is referred to a tertiary care facility). Health care has a rather complex industry structure, caused by the provider-payer-patient triangle. For example, the same hospital episode has several "customers" depending on the point of view; the physician, the payer, and the health care recipient. There are chains of payers: A company contracts with an HMO, which in turn contracts with a hospital, which in turn contracts with physicians. A further complicating factor is the degree of regulation and legislation that concerns health care.

New entrants consist of HMOs, PPOs, "urgicenters," physician group practices, and so forth. Actually, HMOs have existed for twenty years, but they represent a relatively new entrant into the health care arena. Substitute products are wellness centers, health spas, holistic practitioners, improved life-styles.

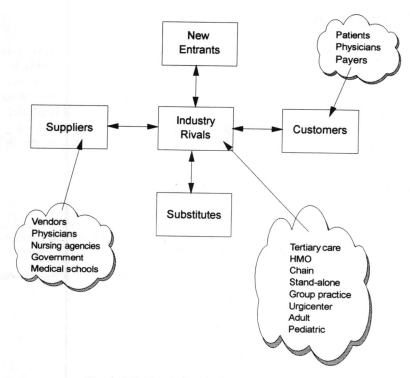

Figure 2.2 Five Factors model for hospitals.

Some readers may object to this mechanistic, "competitive" approach to an area that deals with life and death, and which at times can demonstrate incredible charity and altruism. There are two responses to this objection: (1) Health care is an economic transaction—providers are reimbursed for their services; and (2) even not-for-profit hospitals need to earn excess revenues over expenses. The regulation of health care has created a need to manage resources like a profit-oriented company. No organization can survive without funding sources. A for-profit hospital obtains funding by issuing stock or obtaining loans. The profit it makes goes to repay the stock and loans, to cover expenses, and to build up a war chest for new capital projects—buildings, equipment, systems, and so forth. Not-for-profit hospitals have similar funding concerns. If funding comes from local government, the hospital must worry about the taxing authority's providing enough money. If it does not come from government, then loans must be obtained from external sources. The hospital must earn excess profits over expenses in order to pay back these loans, and to fund new capital projects.

Generic Strategies

In order to maintain their leverage within their industry segment, hospitals have shown a variety of strategies, summarized in Table 2.1. This table shows the range of possibilities. Any one hospital will use only a subset of them, based on its generic strategy. The best way to discuss generic strategy is with a matrix (see Figure 2.3). According to this model, a company can compete on the basis of price or differentiation. In the former case, the primary reason for purchasing the product is the price; in

Table 2.1 Strategies vis-à-vis the Five Factors

Industry component	Hospital response
Suppliers	• They form buyer consortiums. These economies of scale enable them to obtain price concessions from suppliers. • They provide physician incentives, such as equipment or practice management services. • They develop programs to reduce their dependence on nursing agencies that provide higher-priced nurses whose performance is inferior to that of in-house staff.
Customers	• They analyze the profitability of market segments, and try to balance the "mix" of payers. This includes government patients (Medicaid/Medicare) and uninsured patients. • In a related move, they set up marketing data bases to better understand their market segments. • They add value to their existing products. They provide a new "service" orientation by streamlining reservation processes, personalizing menus, setting up patient relation departments, providing easier access to the facility. • They develop new products, including new surgical procedures. • They perform "forward integration," by acquiring insurance companies.
Industry Rivals	• Product differentiation. • Product focus. • Cost accounting. • Productivity management. • Substitutes: Capitated programs. • High-technology equipment. • Formation of chains. • They introduce new organizational structures.
Substitutes	• Expand their product lines to include the substitutes. An example of this would be the formation of an in-house wellness clinic. Another example would be AMI's relationship with the Pritikin clinics.
New entrants	• Formation of chains. • Introduction of high-priced technology.
Internally	• Internal operating efficiencies.

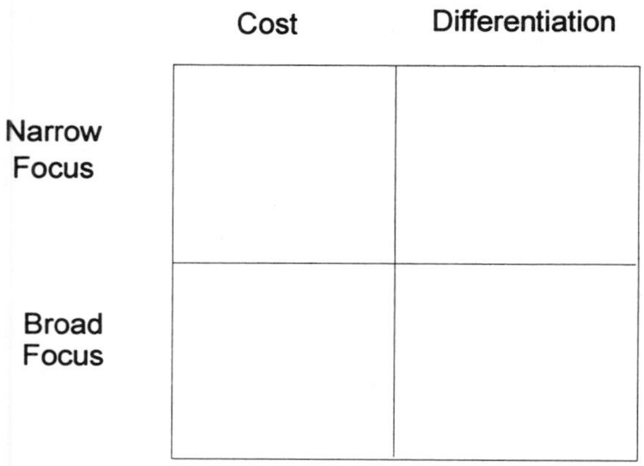

	Cost	Differentiation
Narrow Focus		
Broad Focus		

Figure 2.3 Generic strategy model. (Adapted from Michael Porter, *Competitive Advantage*.)

the latter, the product commands a higher price because it is perceived to have extra "value": inherent quality, extra service features, convenience of distribution channel, extra information, the latest style, etc. Within this framework of price versus differentiation, a company chooses to have either a narrow focus or a broad focus. This refers to the market segments that it pursues. They are frequently defined in socioeconomic or demographic terms.

It is dangerous to adopt a mixed strategy—one that does not fall into one of the four cells in Figure 2.3. This is because a company is run in very different ways, depending on its generic strategy. Kmart clearly has a very different generic strategy from Macy's. Their business processes are different: marketing, sales, inventory control, and so forth. Honda set up a new organization to sell the Acura because they were in a different segment—they were competing against Mercedes and BMW. The Cartier customer probably will not feel comfortable shopping at Zale's, and vice versa.

This model works best for the consumer-goods industry, but it also applies to hospitals. One could object that this model does not account for the physician-patient relationship, for the fact that health care is frequently a matter of life and death, and for the fact that the product is much more complex. Nevertheless, Figure 2.4 presents a classification that has much validity. A VA hospital serves a clearly defined population, and it does not attract its patients on the basis of differentiation. Price is the dominant factor. A county hospital is another kind of public hospital, with the same cost focus, but with a broad population—anyone can go there to get treated. A suburban hospital most likely will compete by differentiating itself for a defined segment—for example, those people

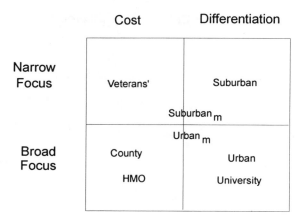

Figure 2.4 Hospital types by generic strategy.

who live in the suburbs and who have private insurance and/or Medicare. The university hospital attracts patients because it is differentiated by its expertise and diversity. Even though university hospitals, since they are teaching hospitals, may provide much free care, this does not mean that they are positioning themselves as low-cost providers. Their cost structure is counter to that. They have much expensive high-tech equipment, high staff-to-patient ratios, extra tests, and uncommon, expensive procedures. In addition, they have to use their charges to fund their teaching and research programs.

Many suburban and urban hospitals are pursuing a "mixed" strategy (located in the middle of Figure 2.4). They mix their focus by accepting both Medicare and private-pay patients; they do not differentiate themselves; they have targeted mixed market segments. Some of these categories overlap. An HMO may be either urban or suburban. A county hospital may also be a teaching hospital. With the exception of the government hospitals, any may belong to a chain, and any may be for-profit.

One's generic strategy affects one's business processes. If one took administrative processes common across all hospitals, such as registration, billing, purchasing, inventory control, discharge planning, and marketing, one would find great differences, depending on the generic strategy of the hospital. Clearly, a suburban hospital that accepts only private-pay patients will do registration, billing, and marketing differently from a county hospital, which has many indigent patients. On the clinical side as well there are differences. HMOs have a different attitude towards redundant tests than do physician-owned hospitals. HMOs also do referrals differently, showing more restraint.

Within its generic strategy, each hospital competes against its segment rivals, pursuing various initiatives to maintain or increase its leverage over the segment's components. A strategy that is appropriate for one type of hospital would not be appropriate for a hospital associated with a medical school. Even teaching hospitals compete. They hire the best clinicians to attract referrals from all over the world.

Many of these initiatives require information systems support. Once again, the number and types of information systems employed by a hospital will depend on its generic strategy and on the specific way it wishes to impact the structural components of its segment.

Use of Information Systems

The Five Factors model can also be applied to information systems. It helps to illuminate those strategic leverage points where information systems can be used to alter or reinforce the structure of the industry to a hospital's advantage. The idea that IS can provide a competitive edge was formally and widely articulated beginning in the mid 1980s. Before that, systems had been used strategically, but there were few formalized models and supporting theories.

In order to respond to these competitive factors, hospitals have developed different types of information systems. They have used information technology to establish better delivery of supplies, to lock in physicians, to get leverage over payers (optimization of reimbursement), to lock in patients (telemarketing), to differentiate their services (ICU system), and to raise barriers for new entrants. This will be discussed in greater detail in subsequent chapters. Table 2.2 summarizes the growth of information systems by the industry phases. In general, before the 1980s, information systems were used mostly to achieve internal efficiencies in billing, materials management, and in the operations of ancillaries. Very little was done to achieve new linkages with the suppliers and customers, or to radically redesign internal business processes. This changed in the mid 1980s with advances in networking and systems integration.

Other Industries

Application of the Five Factors model to other industries can be very enlightening for people who have worked only in the health care industry. There are common structural themes that recur from industry to industry. They include government (regulation and deregulation), extrinsic events (disasters, demographic trends), supplier/customer restructuring (formation of cartels and purchasing groups), and internal restructuring (the strategic moves of individual companies, such as consolidation or expansion). When structural changes occur, companies must change their behavior in order to survive. This behavior could be any business process.

Table 2.2 Information Systems by Industry Phase

Industry phase	Information systems vs. Five Factors
1945–1965 Gov't-sponsored growth; supply emphasized; other aspects of industry remain relatively traditional.	Suppliers: Customers: Computers used very little. Entrants: Internal:
1965–1973 Medicare/Medicaid introduced; access now emphasized; government paid—privately provided. Significant groups not included (poor, children). Health care becomes a big business.	Suppliers: Electronic submittal of orders to vendors. Customers: Entrants: Internal: Efficiencies in billing and collection; efficiencies in A/P.
1973–1983 Costs grow; disenchantment on many fronts; U.S. loses some competitiveness, goes off gold standard; for-profit hospitals emerge. Chains emerge. CON introduced.	Suppliers: Customers: Entrants: Internal: Efficiencies in medical records abstracting; efficiencies in ancillary depts (especially with charge capture).
1983–1991 Disenchantment grows. DRGs introduced. Emphasis on cost (then quality). Hospital profits decrease dramatically, but costs grow.	Suppliers: Linkages with physician offices. Customers: Electronic submittal of claims. Entrants: ICU systems are a barrier. Internal: DRG efficiencies; departmental efficiencies through "niche" systems; cost accounting.
1991– Universal dissatisfaction; National practitioner data base. All constituents agree that health care must be changed fundamentally. More systemic view of problems; threat of greater gov't involvement; combined emphasis on cost + quality + satisfaction.	Suppliers ⎫ Customers ⎬ Systems can be used to support process redesign Entrants ⎪ and restructuring of Internal ⎭ relationships.

One of the critical business processes is data management. You have to know who your customers are; you have to know what your products (and costs) are; you have to understand the quality of your product; you have to know what your markets are; you have to know the status of your assets and resources. Examples of obsoleted information systems abound in industries such as aerospace manufacturing, banking, consumer goods, air travel, and petroleum.

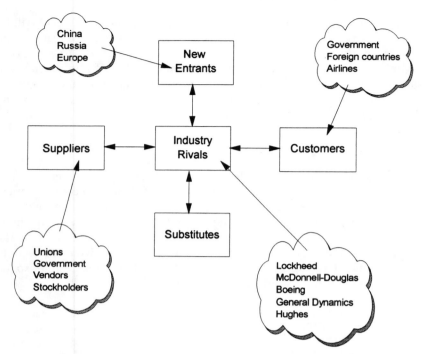

Figure 2.5 Aerospace manufacturing.

Aerospace Manufacturing

Aerospace manufacturing is characterized by relatively few powerful customers, large capital costs, vulnerability to cyclical downturns, and heavy government regulation, due in great part to the fact that the government is one of the largest customers. (See Figure 2.5.) Significant change was introduced into the industry when the government changed its payment policies from cost-plus to fixed-bid. At one time, aersopace companies could incur cost overruns and still have a guaranteed profit margin. When this ended, these companies had to change the way they estimated the cost of their systems initially, and then how they managed the costs of ongoing development. Once again, their information systems did not support this new way of running their business.

Aereospace is complicated in another way. It is really two different businesses—one that deals with the government and another that deals with private airlines. Each has its own criteria for successful management. One could argue that they require different generic strategies.

A greater dislocation has been caused by the end of the cold war, and the concomitant reduction in the defense budget. This will have a huge

(accompanying)

structural impact on the aerospace manufacturing industry. There will be exits from the industry, as well as significant mergers. Companies that remain in the industry will be faced with a dilemma: How does an organization convert from producing military products to producing consumer products? There has to be a major change in culture and processes. The situation is further complicated by new entrants such as Russia and China. Russia too has unused manufacturing capacity.

Banking

Deregulation in the early 1980s caused bank margins to contract. The rates banks could pay on deposits were deregulated, so they could compete for new deposits based on higher rates and additional product features. Unfortunately, there was a risk. Many loan types were fixed rate, meaning that the net income from them was reduced by the higher cost of the money to make them. Other nonbank organizations were allowed to perform some banking activities. Restrictions on how banks could expand geographically were also lifted. (See Figure 2.6).

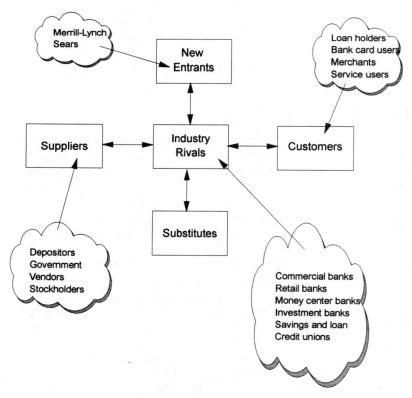

Figure 2.6 Banking.

This resulted in various types of strategic responses: (1) consolidation of facilities, (2) growth through merger and acquisitions, (3) increase in service/convenience, (4) introduction of new banking products, (5) change of cost structure, such as flattening management hierarchies, (6) use of retail techniques, such as advertising and periodic special "sales."

In addition to changing their business processes, banks also needed new types of data. They needed to obtain a consolidated view of each customer and each product line. Unfortunately, their systems architecture did not support this. Each time a bank introduced a new product, it developed a new computer-based delivery system.

Air Travel

The Airline Deregulation Act of 1978 caused significant change in the airline industry. Under regulation, the government subsidized many routes (product lines) that would otherwise have been unprofitable. This ended, creating uncertainty for profit margins. The government also brought down barriers to entry, making it easier to establish and abandon routes. A company could start up business by offering flights that connected as few as two cities (see Figure 2.7). This resulted in both consolidation and

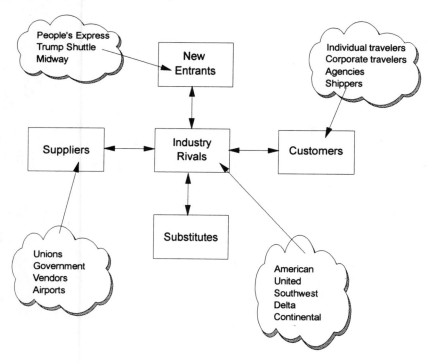

Figure 2.7 Air travel.

expansion. Existing airlines merged, and new airlines appeared. (The latest trend, however, is toward more consolidation.) Airlines significantly changed their distribution channels, moving to a "hub-and-spoke" arrangement. Product differentiation was done through reservations systems and features such as frequent-flyer miles.

There was also a significant effect on information systems. It became important to know what the load factor was, and what was the price elasticity of demand. Prices could change daily. It was important to know the impact of competitors' price changes on demand and profit. The source for much competitive data was the reservation system. Airlines that lacked a reservation system were at a significant disadvantage.

Petroleum

The petroleum industry had a built-in profit margin until the first gas crisis of 1973–1974. Much investment had been made on the assumption of a particular price of gas. Before the Arab oil embargo of 1973, oil price and supply was controlled by major oil companies in the West. Prices were kept low, and supply was assured. When the Arabs took control, the price went from three dollars to ten dollars per barrel overnight. Over the next eight years, the U.S. government attempted to regulate the oil

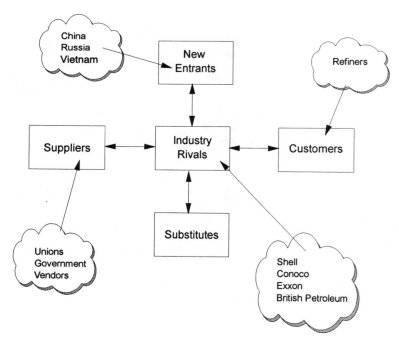

Figure 2.8 Petroleum.

company profits by setting price and allocation controls. This created both high prices and shortages at the same time (see Figure 2.8).

Other Industries

The Japanese have restructured the automotive and consumer electronics industries through their focus on the value-added provided by each process in the business. This has resulted in the movement to total quality, just-in-time inventories, and group problem solving. They all point to the nature of the problem: America has an engineering problem. When an industry changes, one has to reengineer the processes that provide value to the institution or the client, or remove these processes as obsolete. Health care professionals should study other industries for insights about the structural changes occurring in health care.

3
Health Care Information Systems

Over time, health care information systems have evolved, moving through several different phases of technology. These phases roughly correspond to the phases of the health care industry outlined in Table 2.2 in the previous chapter. In addition, one can also observe an evolution in the way that hospitals conceptualize and manage information systems.

History

In the three decades since 1960 there have been several generations of health care information systems technology.[1] This is presented in Table 3.1, which tracks both the technical and the strategic evolution.

First Generation: Early 1960s–Mid 1970s

Two events stand out within this period: the passage of Medicare and the appearance of the IBM 360/370 line of mainframe computers. The first applications of these computers were mostly patient-care oriented, not concerned with administrative functions. The goal was to improve patient care and the productivity of the care givers. Such systems were expensive, and were developed and used by large hospitals (several major vendor systems trace their roots back to this evolution: IBM's PCS product came from a system developed at the Duke University School of Medicine; Spectrum's Omega product is based on the Stonybrook system, which in turn is a derivative of PCS). The first vendors included Lockheed (now

---

[1] For the details of individual vendors and applications, see Richard Sneider, *Management Guide to Health Care Information Systems*, Rockville, MD: Aspen Publishers, 1987.

Table 3.1 Health Care Information Systems by Industry Phase

Industry phase	Data	Technology
1945–1965 Government-sponsored growth.	Manual. No DRG entity.	Almost no information technology.
1965–1973 Medicare/Medicaid introduced.	GL and AP view of data. Patients are viewed as "accounts."	Mainframes. Stand-alone. No standards.
1973–1983 Disenchantment on many fronts—CON.	Patients still viewed as accounts. Utilization data. Profitability reporting.	Minicomputers, PCs. DBMS on mainframe.
1983–1991 DRGs introduced.	Data collection dictated by external organizations. Insurance preauthorization. JCAHO and HCFA data. Cost.	PC networks. PC data bases.
1991– Prospect of national health care.	Product line. Market segment. Demographic segment. Patient viewed as a patient, not an account. New emphasis on enterprise data.	PC networks and data bases. Artificial intelligence. Data interchange.

TDS), McDonnell Douglas (now AMEX), and IBM. Others included Burroughs, HELP, PROMIS, and Meditech. The technology was predominantly mainframe and centralized, with isolated uses of minicomputers, which started to spread in the early 1970s.

Technology is always undergoing change.

Second Generation: Mid 1970s–Early 1980s

Two events mark this: the passage of Certificate of Need legislation, and the appearance of minicomputers. Certificate of Need marks the government's perception that health care expenditures need to be controlled. Minicomputers provide greater opportunities for departmental control. (At the same time, they also provide opportunities for improved and accelerated charge capture.) The next wave of information systems contained applications that supported financial operations, such as charge capture and order entry. This coincided with increased complexity in billing and reimbursement. Increased miniaturization of hardware, as well as its reduced price, allowed smaller hospitals to purchase their own computers. Affordability was an issue. Programming methods were very rigid. Vendors included HBO (with its Medpro product), SMS (Action), and McDonnell Douglas (HDC). Minicomputers were used widely.

During this stage, technology was undergoing other changes, beyond the introduction of minicomputers. In the late 1970s and early 1980s there was a new emphasis on data bases. These systems had more flexibility in screen and report design. This period was characterized by increased miniaturization of systems, and so, many departmental and niche systems sprang up. These systems were either stand-alone or loosely interfaced, but integration was a secondary issue. Low-cost financial systems were developed for hospitals with less than 200 beds. The second-generation products, in turn, expanded into patient-care applications.

Third Generation: Early 1980s–1991

Two events mark the beginning of this period: passage of DRG legislation and the introduction of the personal computer (PC). The concept of prospective payment signaled the need for new technology or new use of existing technology. Prospective payment, in theory, forced hospitals to behave more competitively, requiring that they manage costs, product lines, and markets, for the first time. The major technological feature was niche functionality on PCs and LANs. Towards the end of this period the need for integration and standards came to the forefront. The major vendor theme was shakeout, consolidation, and the appearance of new vendors.

- IBM and Baxter entered into a joint venture, which subsumed the former Omega and Delta products. Baxter sold its Sigma product (formerly Compucare) back to its previous owners.
- AMEX acquired Saint and McDonnell Douglas.
- GTE acquired Intermountain.
- AMI spun off PHS as an independent entity.
- SMS took Spirit (a combination of Computer Synergy and Action) and turned it into Allegra, and created a separate division, Turnkey Systems Division, to market this product.
- 3M acquired the LDS system.
- New entrants were PHAMIS and Gerber Alley.

During this period, many vendors had to "re-architect" their product, in particular, to make it more "open." For example, HBO moved its Star product from Maxi Mumps to C. Other examples were SMS (Independence), McDonnell Douglas (IHS). TDS was a pioneer in integration. At this time Local Area Networks (LANs) were developing. As the old guard vendors underwent restructuring, new niche vendors were proliferating. Sophisticated systems for hospitals could be developed on microcomputers.

In this period, the momenturn for adoption of standards began to gain strength. These included HL7, MEDIX, and the MIB, as well as X12. It also included operating systems, networks, and file management systems. Ethernet was becoming the standard for backbone networks. Vendors were moving away from proprietary operating systems and were using accepted third-party data base management systems. More and more tools were available for data management. Some data base management systems had query languages that could access other vendors' data bases to provide an integrated view of the data.

A few vendors continued their proprietary stance. Notable among them was Meditech. This worked well in less complex environments, or where users do not have high data requirements. However, toward the end of this period even Meditech had begun to move toward more open systems.

Fourth Generation: Starting in 1991

A new generation is beginning to appear, even though the trends of the previous generation have not been played out completely. There are several factors influencing this phase: (1) the government's announcement that it intends to collect electronic data on quality of care, (2) the increase in the connectivity of networks, (3) the ability of data base management systems to span multiple networks and multiple data bases and, (4) the growth of standards. The imminent prospect of some form of national health care and the shift towards centers of excellence, managed care, and consolidation, will play a role.

Telecommunications vendors like Ameritech, GTE, and Atlantic Bell are acquiring health care software vendors, sitting up networks for EDI, and constructing regional data bases. Systems integrators like Perot Systems are becoming more prominent in health care. This period will see the broad use of technologies that are incipient in the Third Generation, but which foster integration. These include expert systems, voice recognition, voice synthesis (talking data bases), and electronic imaging (the electronic chart). If the Third Generation can be viewed as the period in which connectivity tools were developed, then the Fourth Generation can be viewed as the time when hospitals begin to learn how to use these tools. That is, with expert systems, the information system is inextricably bound and interwoven to the business processes. It must be used. With the electronic chart, all patient data, no matter what the modality—voice, X-ray, cinema image, text, numbers, waveforms, images of documents—will be computerized.

This current period will see continued vendor restructuring. HBO, which spun off its mainframe business into a separate company, has reversed this decision and reunited it with its Star line. Ferranti has gone out of business. Keane is growing through acquisition. TDS has been sold Gerber Alley has been acquired by American Express. More and more vendors are entering into cross-marketing arrangements as users demand more functionality and integration. The vendors that will prosper will be those that have paid attention to architecture, standards, and tools. They will be able to incorporate new technology faster and more easily than other vendors, to meet increasing hospital demands for integration and end-user tools.

Technology Adoption (Leads and Lags)

The previous discussion shows that evolving business requirements (dictated by economics, social forces, consolidation of buyers and/or sellers) frequently create a need for new technology. The data bases need to be changed; new functions need to be added to existing programs; systems need to be integrated, and so forth. The previous discussion also shows that it takes years for vendors to replace their obsoleted systems— anywhere from five to ten years. This gives rise to a "lead-lag" situation, whereby technology is always trailing business events. This concept is shown in Figure 3.1. In this model, the vertical axis represents the cumulative number of hospitals that realize the existence of a business need and react to it. The horizontal axis represents time. The curve itself is a traditional growth curve. Initially, few hospitals realize that the industry structure has changed. Over time, more hospitals realize that a structural change has occurred, and they move to react to it. This movement continues at an accelerating rate. At point X the growth of hospitals changing starts to decelerate, as most hospitals have already taken steps to adapt. At the tail of the curve are those hospitals that have not been able to change, and whose survival is in question.

A given information system has an underlying model, which reflects the

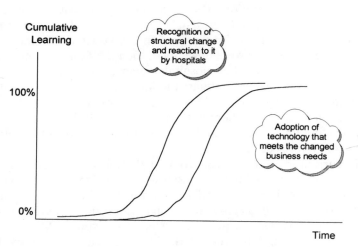

Figure 3.1 Technology lag factor.

structure of an industry at some point in time. The challenge for the hospital is to choose systems whose underlying model is relatively up-to-date. Each generation of information systems contains a certain technology, with inherent capabilities and limitations, and it is written with a generic model of the industry at a given point in time in mind. The second curve in Figure 3.1 shows this lagging effect of technology. Even those hospitals that recognize the structural change and hence the need for new systems, will have trouble obtaining new systems. Those hospitals situated on the right-hand tail of the curve are doomed to having obsolete systems.

For example, in 1984, when diagnosis related groups (DRGs) were introduced, hospitals had an urgent need for information systems that allowed all of a patient's accounts to be associated, both inpatient and outpatient. However, hospitals still had an older generation of systems, and vendors were still selling that older generation. Because of technology restrictions, and because of an older view of the industry, these systems could not easily support the new business reality.

It was stated that each figure represents a learning curve. The hospitals learn about the structure of the industry; they also learn about the management of the technology (discussed later).

Impacting the Industry through Information Technology

Instead of using information systems to simply react to structural changes, it is possible to use them to turn these changes to the hospital's advantage, or even to influence the form of the changes themselves. This has been argued by such authorities as Michael Porter, who has applied the Five Factors model to analyze the opportunities to use information technology to alter the balance of power in an industry segment. Figure 3.2 shows the structural characteristics from the IT point of view. In general, information systems can be used to lock in suppliers by implementing electronic linkages, to lock in customers through electronic linkages and technology value-added, to do product innovation, and to reshape the company through process redesign, enabled by networks, data bases, and groupware. In particular, hospitals have done the following:

Hospital-Supplier

1. Hospitals are trying to tie physicians more closely to their facility by allowing them to preregister a patient, order tests and view results, call up the medical record, do trending, and so forth. Some hospitals also provide practice management features through their information system. The net result is to ensure a reliable supply of patients with a certain type of insurance.

Study
This
*

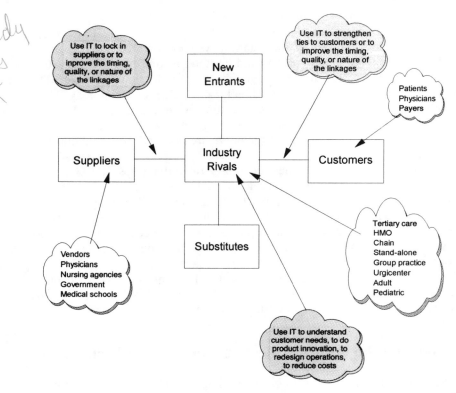

Figure 3.2 IT and the structural characteristics of the healthcare industry.

2. Hospitals have established electronic links with their inventory suppliers for faster response time, more accurate orders, and reduced holding costs (although this could also be viewed as a case of the supplier locking in the hospital).

3. Hospitals can use electronic linkages to provide data on quality and utilization to regulators, in an effort to influence regulatory decisions.

Hospital-Customer

1. A hospital might use IT to integrate different levels of facilities, such as acute-care facility, skilled nursing facility, long-term care facility, and clinic. This makes it easier for a given customer to stay within the hospital's system.

2. Electonic data interchange can be used to provide quality, cost, satisfaction, and utilization data to employers and insurers, in order to influence their choice of care provider.

3. IT can be used to support telemarketing activities, to channel potential patients to certain hospital services.

Intra-Segment Rivalry

1. Provide added value to the product: Many hospitals are upgrading their registration systems to provide more hotel-like services.

2. Use IT to understand the market segments and customer needs, through the creation of marketing data bases.

3. Use IT for product differentiation. Use IT to deliver the product faster, more accurately, with less expense; or at a different time or place; or deliver it with a higher information content.

4. React quickly: Many hospitals have installed Cost Accounting systems. In very competitive industries, it is important to know your costs so that you can react quickly to moves by the competition and the regulators.

5. Use IT for research on product innovation. This mostly applies to hospitals affiliated with medical schools.

6. Use IT to facilitate structural changes, such as formation of a chain to respond to industry consolidation.

Hospital-New Entrant

Create barriers for new entrants and substitutes: expensive integrated information systems.

When a hospital adopts a strategic attitude toward information systems it needs to understand how it ranks vis-à-vis its peers with regard to the use of information technology. One technique is to use a "Strategic Grid," shown in Figure 3.3. On this grid, the X axis represents the "marketing intensity" of IT for a particular industry. The Y axis represents the "manufacturing intensity" of IT. Each varies from "high" to "low." For nonhospitals, marketing activities have to do with product planning, selection, purchase, and after-sales service. Manufacturing activities concern the production of the product: the design, manufacturing, assembly, testing, and inventory activities.

For a hospital, marketing activities would include research for product innovation; marketing medical services to physicians, patients, insurers, and other hospitals; admitting and discharge; patient service representatives; a service number to call for questions about bills and physicians. The marketing information systems could include physician access systems, marketing data bases, special admit cards, patient correspondence data bases, reservation systems, and so forth.

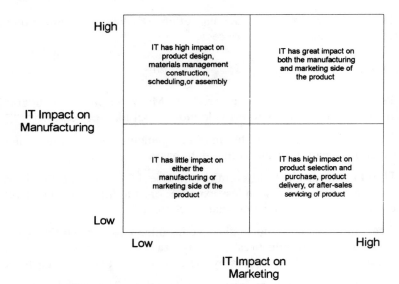

Figure 3.3 Strategic grid for IT. (Adapted from James Cash et al., *Corporate Information Systems Management: Text and Cases.*)

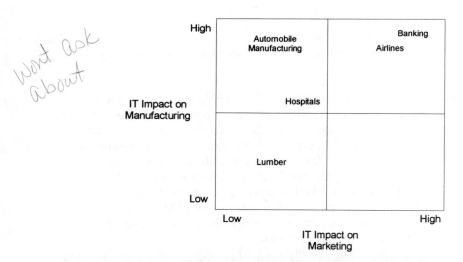

Figure 3.4 Strategic grid for several industries. (Adapted from James Cash et al., *Corporate Information Systems Management: Text and Cases.*)

For a hospital, the manufacturing activities would include all the ancillary departments, nursing care (both floor and ICU), surgery, and so forth. The manufacturing information systems would include: orders, care plans, lab, radiology, surgery scheduling, inventory control, patient monitoring, and so forth.

IT marketing and manufacturing intensity vary from industry to industry (and within a particular industry). Industry differences are shown in Figure 3.4. This figure shows that banking and airlines, traditionally, are much more intense in their use of information technology than are hospitals. For example, banking relies heavily on check readers, digital imaging of checks, electronic funds transfer, ATMs, and, increasingly, home banking terminals. The IT intensity of hospitals is changing, however, as evidenced by the increasing installation of ICU systems and physician-access modules. Automobile manufacturers use just-in-time electronic inventories, robots, and CAD-CAM, resulting in high manufacturing IT intensity, but they do not use information technology as heavily to support/influence the buying decision. Health care has trailed other industries in its use of information technology for several reasons: the size of the average hospital, the structure of the industry, and competitive factors.

Within the health care industry itself, the intensity of information technology use varies considerably. This is illustrated in Figure 3.5, which contains several different segments of the health care industry.

1. *University*: A large university hospital, in an urban setting, treating a mix of insured and uninsured patients, will have high manufacturing

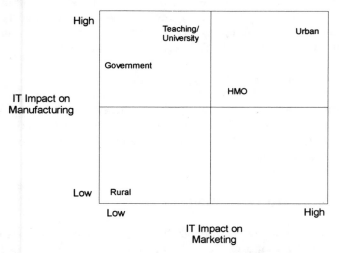

Figure 3.5 Strategic grid for hospitals.

intensity for its information systems. They might include an ICU information system, an OR system, an ER system, links with other tertiary care facilities. On the other hand, its marketing intensity is not so high. The university gets many referrals. It is a prestige item for doctors to have admitting privileges there.

2. *Rural*: A small rural hospital with no close competition and with forty beds does not need a high-availability patient-care system, nor does it need extensive marketing system support. The rural hospital will be relatively low in both manufacturing and marketing intensity. It has a guaranteed market, and the more complex cases are transported to other hospitals, which possess more technology.

3. *Urban*: A large urban acute-care facility in a competitive city, competing for private-pay patients and trying to project an image, will be high in both manufacturing and marketing intensity. It will have the latest in ICU information systems, and it will pay particular attention to its marketing data base, and the speed and accuracy of its reservation and admitting system. Its billing system will be fast and accurate. It caters to the private-pay market and needs to do everything it can to retain its clientele, including its physicians.

Treat Primary care

4. *HMO*: An HMO in a large urban area, might possibly be lower in both manufacturing and marketing intensity than the urban hospital in Figure 3.5. This is because the HMO has a committed clientele and because it is interested in prevention rather than intervention, contracting out the more complicated surgical cases. (Prevention)

County Hosp.

5. *Government*: A county hospital, in an urban setting, treating many indigent patients, will be relatively high in the manufacturing intensity of its information systems, and very low in the marketing intensity. It treats many difficult cases, but they are indigent. It is a sad fact, but true. Its clientele will not switch. They have nowhere else to go.
They way Private Paying Patients

The hospital must create a grid and plot itself vis-à-vis its competitors to determine how it ranks within its industry segment. If it lags its competitors, but has the same generic strategy, it will probably have to invest additional money in its information systems. Alternatively, it may be able to develop a different strategy than its competitors, one that does not require the same IT intensity.

Approaches to IT Management

It is not enough to think strategically about the business and systems. It is also not enough to introduce modern technology. There is a third element, the strategic management of IT, and this represents another learning

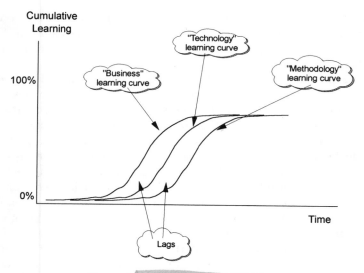

Figure 3.6 Methodology lag factor.

curve. This additional learning curve is illustrated in Figure 3.6, and is called the "methodology factor." The second curve represents the organization's learning about the given technology: how to physically install it; how to use it and maintain it; how to integrate it with other technologies. The third curve represents the management of IT within an organizational setting. IT management is widely misunderstood. Non-IT staff think it is the arcane activities of systems programming and hardware maintenance (curve two). In actuality, IT management is a set of general management activities that just happen to be performed within a technical context. They include items such as justification and cost-benefit analysis; prioritization; planning and budgeting; standards, policies, and procedures; reward systems, and so on. These are activities performed in every area of the hospital.

There are three generic approaches to the management of IT, called "Eras." They are illustrated in Table 3.2. The categories to be examined are: administration, user, and justification. The category of "Administration" includes the activities of planning, funding, prioritizing, operation,

Table 3.2 Generic Approaches to IT Management

	Administration	User	Justification
Era I	Regulated monopoly	Department	Cost
Era II	Free market	Individual	Individual effectiveness
Era III	Regulated free market	Enterprise	Achievement of strategic goals

Source: James Cash et al., *Corporate Information Systems Management: Text and Cases.*

development, and support of systems. The category of "User" refers to the identity of the end user of a given system. The category of "Justification" refers to the type of cost-benefit analysis that is performed for a system.

In Era I, IT is administered centrally, and has been called a "regulated monopoly." This means that a centralized IT organization makes most of the decisions about information systems, for example, what funds will be allocated to what projects. In this approach, IT planning is generally done separately from strategic business planning. Systems are developed for individual departments and functions, on a vertical basis. The justification focuses on cost reduction and other business efficiencies. The technology is typically centralized mainframes, or large shared host computers. In health care, probably more than any other industry, these centralized hosts were "shared systems," that is, hospitals dialed in for remote access to a shared host. The applications were at the operational level for the business services and finance departments: patient accounting and registration. There was a monopoly on the data. Data for management decision making was inaccessible. The hospital end user was highly dependent on the system administrator for everything.

In Era II, IT management is more decentralized, and has been called a "free market." Individual departments do their own funding, planning, prioritization, and, in many cases, installation, of information systems. Equipment standards and software decisions are no longer dictated by the Information Systems Department. The needs of individual users are emphasized because many professional activities are not supported well under Era I. Thus, the justification shifts from "efficiency" to "effectiveness." Data is required to make the individuals within the ancillary departments more effective. Applications are tailored more for the individual, or for niches within a department. Examples are nurse scheduling, QA, encoders. A typical scenario is for the end user of a centralized host to purchase a PC, attach it emulating a dumb terminal, and download data to his PC for purposes of analysis and processing, which could not be done on the centralized system.

Era III is characterized by a balance in the management of IT, and has been called a "regulated free market." There is a shared responsibility—among IT, general management, and end users—for the planning, funding, prioritization, development, and operation. The user of a system is no longer an individual but the enterprise, or at least a horizontal layer of the organization, spanning several departments. The justification for a system is that it contributes to the strategic goals of the enterprise. People are free to make purchase and access decisions within corporate standards, which include hardware/software standards, connectivity standards, data base standards, and security standards. Examples are: buying any system, as long as it conforms to the HL7 standard; LANs that are attached to a backbone network; multiple niche applications that share the same data base.

There is a correlation between IT management approach and industry stage and technology. This is illustrated in Table 3.3. In general, Era I was used with mainframe computers, at a time when there was less competition within the health care industry. Era II appeared toward the end of the minicomputer era and the beginning of the PC era, as the government was trying to introduce more competition into health care. Era III has emerged only recently, as networking technology starts to

Table 3.3 Industry Phase and Learning Curves

Industry phase	Business need	Technology	IT management

1945–1965
Government-
  sponsored growth.
	Construction and
	  facilities.
	  Intervention
	  (rather than
	  prevention).
		Mainframe	Era I

1965–1973
Medicare/Medicaid
  introduced.
  Government paid—
  privately provided.
  Significant groups
  not included (poor,
  children).
	Construction and
	  facilities. Billing.
	  Department level.
	  Inpatient
	  orientation.
		Mainframe	Era I

1973–1983
Disenchantment on
  many fronts. U.S.
  goes off gold
  standard. For-profit
  hospitals emerge.
  Chains emerge.
  CON introduced.
	Billing. Marketing.
	  Utilization review.
	  Corporate
	  functions. Capital
	  for acquisitions.
	  Insurance.
		Minicomputers	Era I/II

1983–1991
Disenchantment
  grows. DRGs
  introduced.
  Emphasis on cost
  (then quality).
  Hospital profits
  decrease
  dramatically.
	Prospective
	  utilization review.
	  Concurrent QA.
	  Costing. Inventory
	  control.
	  Management
	  engineering.
	  Emphasis on
	  outpatient.
	  Strategic planning.
		Personal
		  computers
			Era II

1991–
National practitioner
  DB. All
  constituents agree
  that national health
  care must be
  instituted.
	Switch to prevention.
	  Total quality
	  management.
	  HMO style of
	  management.
	  Consolidation of
	  facilities.
		Networking	Era III

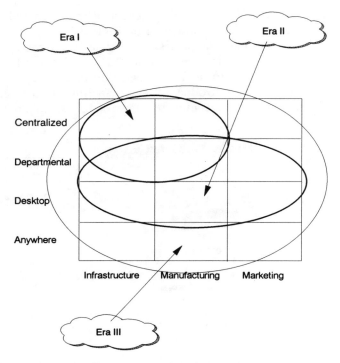

Figure 3.7 Eras versus value chain and organization.

dominate, and as global changes face the health care industry (along with global competition for the United States). It is easy to see how the business needs drive the technology needs, and how the technology drives IT management needs. Thus, there arises the concept of "fit." There is a certain alignment among business need, technology, and IT management. The better the fit, the more competitive the hospital will be. One can find hospitals in which there is misalignment among two or more of the above-mentioned factors: industry phase, business need, technology, and IT management. There are still hospitals that have not fully reacted to the business environment of 1983–1991, even though a new era is dawning. It is still possible to find hospitals trying to force mainframe technology upon a business need that really requires a more responsive technology. It is also possible to find hospitals trying to force Era I onto the management of an environment that has many PCs. These instances of misalignment might be acceptable in a static, noncompetitive environment, but not in an environment that requires a fast response and a linkage between strategic planning and systems planning.

Figure 3.7 shows the relative fit between IT eras and industry situations. On the vertical axis it shows the spread of IT from a centralized environment to a ubiquitous environment. On the horizontal axis it shows three aspects of the business that are supported by IT: infrastructure, manufacturing, and marketing. IT Era I arose at a time when emphasis was on infrastructure and manufacturing using a centralized or departmental framework. It does not work well as the technology moves to the desk top and beyond, out into the world. It also does not work well as more and more of the marketing activities gain IT support.

IT Management Learning Curve

Within a given era, the organization over time learns how to use a given technology. This can be represented by the S-shaped learning curve in Figure 3.8. There are four general phases of learning:

1. *Initiation*: The technology is introduced. This is characterized by caution and analysis. Spread of the technology is slow, as the organization tries to understand its applicability to business problems, as well as its costs and benefits.

2. *Learning Growth*: Explosive growth and loss of control. As the company begins to feel more secure about the technology it launches many development projects, but without having a control infrastructure (which would include project management system, budgets and chargebacks, prioritization mechanisms, cost-benefit analysis, and systems development methodology).

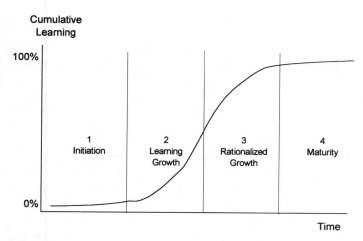

Figure 3.8 Stages of methodology learning. (Adapted from James Cash et al., *Corporate Information Systems Management: Text and Cases*.)

3. *Rationalized Growth*: Control is introduced, in the form of methodologies, project management techniques, organizational structures, budgets, prioritization, and so forth.

4. *Maturity*: The company learns how to manage the technology, and it becomes widespread throughout the enterprise.

In actuality, the curve never flattens out; instead, the organization brings in another technology and moves onto another learning curve. At any given point in time, the hospital is on several different technology curves simultaneously. By 1991, a large hospital will have gone through mainframes, followed by minicomputers, PCs, and LANs. While it is still learning how best to manage mainframes, it adds minicomputers. It is then learning how to manage minicomputers, in addition to learning how to manage the mixed environment. This continues, with subsequent acquisitions of PCs and Local Area Networks, yielding an aggregated learning curve.

The management processes for mainframe technology in the control phase may not be appropriate for a different technology that is in a different stage of evolution.

Mainframe applications had been in existence for many years before professionals proposed commonly accepted ways of consistently analyzing and designing systems. Likewise, data base technology had been in existence for many years before data-driven methodologies became popular. Unfortunately, these methodologies still lag the technologies. Very few vendors practice these methodologies on a wide scale.

Architectures

Beyond technology, the ultimate strategy may be to create an organization that can learn faster than the competitors. This will ensure a faster alignment of technology and IT management with the business needs and a faster perception of the business needs, together with the appropriate organizational structures to address these business needs. Thus, the organization "shrinks" the learning curves and maintains a lead on its competitors as each structural change occurs.

This leads to the concept of "architecture" introduced in Chapter 1. Chapter 1 stated that the book would address four different architectures: Business Architecture, Data Architecture, Technical Architecture, and Control Architecture. In reality, these "architectures" are the result of organizational learning, whereby a hospital explicitly defines and structures its organizational components in response to industry change. Figure 3.9 shows the relation between the learning curves and architectures.

To review, the aspects of these architectures are the following:

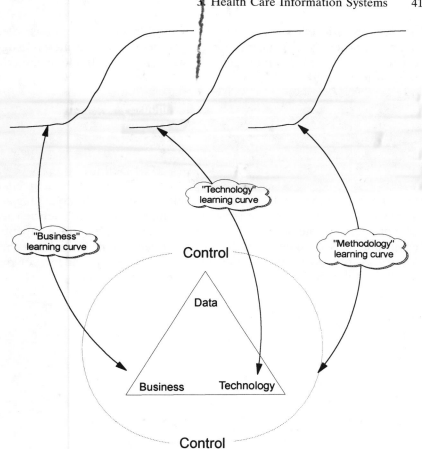

Figure 3.9 Organizational learning and architectures.

1. *Business Architecture*: The process of understanding the structure of the industry and responding to it with the appropriate business processes; the design of these business processes, and their measurement. Examples of business processes are: patient registration, order entry, and so on.

2. *Data Architecture*: Understanding how the data fits together; distributing it in the right way to the interested departments. Integrated data facilitates integration of the organization, which facilitates service and quality.

3. *Technical Architecture*: The data collection and distribution network, including software, hardware, networks, and protocols that they use.

4. *Control Architecture*: The organizations and controls that govern the systems management process. This includes such items as steering com-

mittee, strategic plan, budgets, data ownership policy, top-down commitment, project management methodology, development methodology, capacity planning methodology, change management methodology, service request methodology.

Every hospital has a business architecture and a systems architecture that support its strategic response to its industry segment. Its systems architecture is a blueprint of the business systems and information technology. Its organization consists of business systems, the data that is used by these business systems, and the computer systems that both automate tasks and distribute the data. Finally, there is a control architecture that ensures a fit among all the components. In most hospitals, these architectures have arisen in a rather random fashion, without much planning and analysis. This has caused organizational inefficiencies and deficiencies. The paradigm of the health care industry is changing, and the competitve environment is becoming less forgiving. Organizations must learn their lessons faster; having formal architectures is not only evidence of past learning, but also of readiness to engage in future learning.

4
Business Architecture

GENERAL DISCUSSION

"Business Architecture" refers to the way in which a hospital organizes itself to achieve its strategy. It includes departmental structure, job design, work flows, systems for rewarding and motivating employees, systems for defining and measuring standards of performance, and other organizational entities such as teams, committees, and advisory groups. While strategy is necessary, it is not sufficient; it requires sharp execution in order to succeed. This fact, until fairly recently, has been ignored by many industries, particularly by hospitals. After the strategy has been developed, it must be carried out by organizations and their components: work groups, policies, procedures, skills, work flows, and supporting technology.

As a matter of fact, when one examines the structural characteristics of an industry and the capabilities of one's company, one finds there are only a limited number of strategies available to the company. Many hospitals, when doing strategic planning, will arrive at the same set of strategies. Not all of these hospitals, however, will be successful, and the reason is that many will fail to properly execute an otherwise sound strategy.

Aligning Business Architecture with Strategy

The strategy of a hospital specifies what the hospital will do in order to achieve its long-term goals. It defines where the hospital will compete, and how it will compete, in general. When the hospital develops its strategy, it examines both the external environment (competitors, economics, social trends, industry structure) and the internal environment (hospital structure and performance). As part of its strategy, the hospital defines what aspects of the external environment it will try to affect, as well as what aspects of its internal environment (structure) it will try to affect. This internal structure is the Business Architecture.

At its simplest level, the Business Architecture consists of a series of activities performed by departments and individuals. This book calls these activities "business processes." Business processes range from Accounts Payable to Surgery. Some of them, such as Surgery, provide direct value to the customer, whether patient, insurer, or physician. Other processes exist only to support the delivery of the product, and they provide "internal" value. Among these indirect processes there is a hierarchy of relevance, ranging from Central Supply (less remote) to Accounts Payable (more remote). Each business process is a complex entity, consisting of tasks, people, procedures, equipment, work flows, data flows, standards, controls, and so on. Sometimes the business processes break down, as measured by poor outcomes, low satisfaction, turnover, delays, and so forth. When this happens, the reasons can be complex, and they are to be found in the components of the process.

It is useful to view each business process as contributing a layer of value to the product. Customers place a value on these services according to quality of medical outcome, quality of service, and price. The value of these processes to the customer can be higher or lower, depending on how well they are performed. Once again, the quality of their performance depends on the working of their components: work flows, equipment, training, skills, motivation, policies, and procedures.

It is here that the "architectural" metaphor can be appreciated. When a hospital fails to achieve its strategic objectives, it is because its Business Architecture is not aligned with the strategy. Repairing the Business Architecture is an engineering activity. If the components of the business processes do not fit together, then value is diminished. The value of a skilled surgeon is reduced by a poor schedule or poorly maintained equipment. The value as perceived by the customer is reduced by a confusing admitting process or by an unmotivated housekeeping staff.

Value-Chain Analysis

As previously stated, taken together, the activities of many individuals and many departments create this value for the customer(s). Bit by bit, each activity adds value to the customer. A model for this chain of activities has been widely publicized by Michael Porter. This model distinguishes between those activities that are directly associated with the product and those activities that constitute the hospital's infrastructure. This model is provided in Figure 4.1.

This model was originally developed for manufacturing organizations,

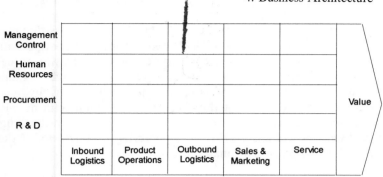

	Inbound Logistics	Product Operations	Outbound Logistics	Sales & Marketing	Service	
Management Control						
Human Resources						Value
Procurement						
R & D						

Figure 4.1 Value chain. (Source: Michael Porter, *Competitive Advantage*.)

which have large, highly developed purchasing and inventory operations, as well as complex logistics to accompany extensive activities in product design, manufacture, and assembly. A sales firm would not be so balanced. In addition, the terms "inbound logistics" and "operations" seem alien to a hospital environment. Nevertheless, this model can provide valuable insights for people who have been involved with health care all their professional lives. Other industries have made much progress in defining the activities in their value chain. For a manufacturing firm, the direct product activities are the following:

Inbound Logistics: Activities such as ordering, receiving, storage, and inventory.
Operations: Product design and manufacturing operations: drilling, cutting, pressing, coating, and so forth. It also concerns assembly as well as the storage of items in process.
Outbound Logistics: Product packing, shipping, and delivery.
Sales and Marketing: Sales and advertising activities, helping the customer with purchase decisions, development of marketing programs, and so on.
Service: Post-sale customer service, including the handling of complaints, follow-up, field-servicing of the items, spares inventory, and so on.

The indirect activities of manufacturing are:

Management Control: The traditional functions of Finance and Accounting, and management reporting, analysis, control, and planning.
Human Resources: The recruitment and retention of qualified staff, management of compensation and benefits.
Procurement: This includes activities such as negotiation of contracts with suppliers.
Technology Development: The research and development function.

In value-chain analysis, one examines areas in the business that can be changed to provide more value to the customer (or to other organizations within the company). The product may be examined narrowly, to determine how to improve its features or delivery; or it can be examined from a broader perspective, looking at the contributions by all the departments. For example, quality checking by Manufacturing means that Assembly will produce fewer defective items. Quality checking by Inbound Logistics will ensure that Manufacturing produces fewer defective items due to substandard materials.

Health Care Value Chain

In health care, Product Operations are Patient Care activities. The patient is the raw material flowing through the hospital. The raw material arrives in one state, and leaves in another state. The patient arrives ill and leaves well (hopefully). While the patient is in the hospital, services are provided to her/him, just as processes are applied to a raw material or semifinished material in manufacturing. Of course, this analogy does not account for the importance of prevention, and for the complexity of

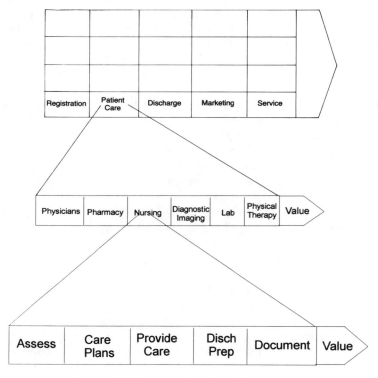

Figure 4.2 Constituent value chains.

the human body. These services include Nursing and all the activities of the ancillary departments. Each activity and department contributes to the overall value, as illustrated in Figure 4.2.

In health care, the activities of the value chain have their own unique characteristics:

1. *Inbound Logistics*: How the patient is acquired and brought into the hospital. This would include physician referrals, transfers from other hospitals, registration, as well as admitting and pre-admitting. This also includes the acquisition of materials.

2. *Patient Care*: Includes traditional ancillary department activities such as Lab, Pharmacy, Radiology, Physical Therapy, and Respiratory Therapy. This also includes the development of new products and services, such as a new technique for closing holes in the heart. It also includes home health care.

3. *Outbound Logistics*: Includes the discharge of the patient and the delivery of the product through distribution channels, such as clinics and home health programs.

4. *Sales and Marketing*: Concerned with the identification and analysis of new markets. This also includes referral programs.

5. *Service*: In manufacturing, this comprises post-sales service; in health care, this comprises post-discharge service. This is an activity that is rapidly changing and expanding. It includes such diverse activities as answering questions about patient bills, the servicing of equipment located in the patient's home, provision of educational materials, and so forth.

Infrastructure activities in health care have greater similarities with those of manufacturing:

Research and Development: This is the basic research done by a medical school that is affiliated with a given hospital. Community hospitals would not have this function, just as not every industrial company has this function.

Figure 4.2 breaks Patient Care into its constituent value chains. The first level consists of physician activities, nursing activities, pharmacy, diagnostic imaging, laboratory, and physical therapy. The second level focuses on nursing activities: assessment, care plans, medical care, help with daily living, and discharge planning. Obviously, the structure and complexity of these value chains are quite different from those of companies in other industries (e.g., manufacturing, distribution, transportation, etc.).

Some hospitals have simpler product operations; others have more complex, comprehensive product operations. For example, a rural adult critical-care hospital has cases that are more uniform and simpler than the cases of a tertiary-care teaching hospital, which might have a product line called "transplants" that includes many services, such as lab tests, surgery, pharmacy, immunology, and physical therapy.

Redesigning the Value Chain

The engineering metaphor can be continued in the concept of "value-added." It is revealing to recall what the Japanese did as they rebuilt their industries in the 1950s and 1960s. In order to enter American markets, they would acquire samples of American products that they desired to manufacture and "reverse engineer" them, disassembling them into their components, analyzing each component to understand how it functioned and what "value" it provided, and redesigning the component to provide greater value.

Each of the nursing activities in Figure 4.3 consists of people, policies, procedures, work flows, equipment, data, and leadership. Each activity

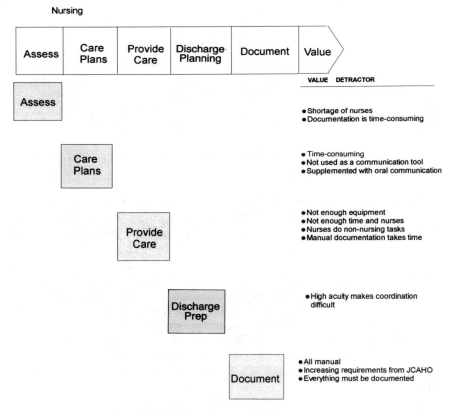

Figure 4.3 Value detractors in the value chain.

must be examined to see how it contributes to the hospital's value-added, and, if there are problems, to see how it can be improved.

The meaning of "value" has changed over time. In general industry, it has undergone an evolution from "good price" to "good price plus quality," and finally to "good price + good quality + fast delivery." At one time, defects were considered to be an unavoidable part of the production process. However, by understanding these processes better, companies are able to improve them and reduce defects.

In health care, this evolution has been a little different. The concept of health care value has gone from "good quality" to "good quality + good price" and finally to "good quality + good price + fast delivery and patient satisfaction." In general industry, the product designers have shifted their focus from how the *company* views the product to how the *customer* views and uses the product. This means examining the customer's value chain. Health care too, if it is to provide value, must

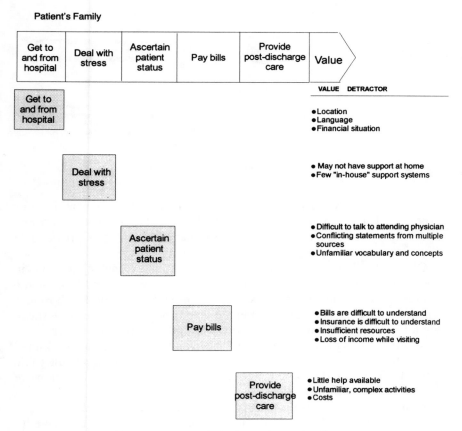

Figure 4.4 Value chain for patient's family.

Physician

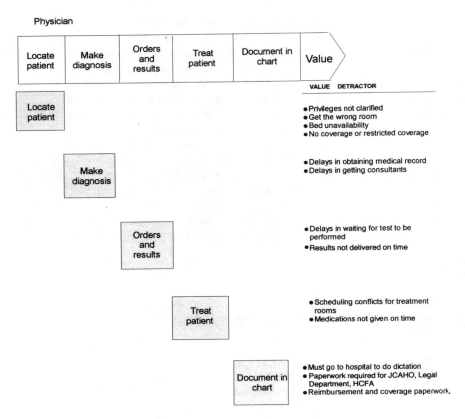

Figure 4.5 Value chain for physician.

look at the value chains of its customers to see how they view and use its products. The hospital's customers include patients, physicians, insurers, and employers. The value chain for the patient's family is provided in Figure 4.4, and for physicians in Figure 4.5.

Obviously, there is close and intense interaction among departments in the care of patients, and this demands analysis. We should look at the interaction of value chains. This interaction is often ignored in hospitals whose culture is department-oriented and whose structure is vertical. Figure 4.6 shows Nursing's interaction with other departments.

Reference was previously made to the evolution of the concept "value" in health care. In particular, the concept of value has come full circle since 1945, when the primary focus was on the construction of more facilities. This is shown below:

1945–1965: Emphasis on increased construction of *facilities*.

1965–1973: Emphasis shifts to *accessibility*, providing coverage to senior citizens and indigent.

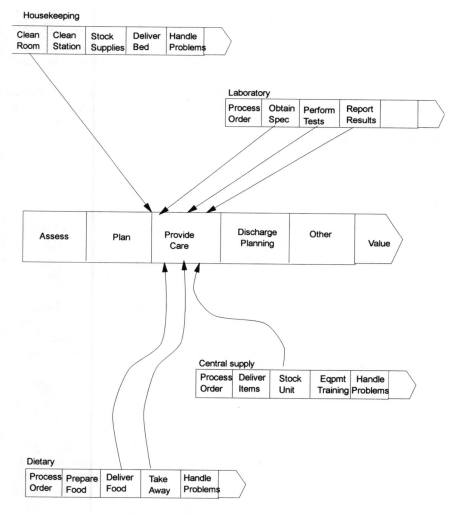

Figure 4.6 Value chain interaction.

1973–1983: Emphasis shifts to *necessity*—is a given facility or piece of equipment really needed?

1983–1991: Emphasis shifts to utilization—is the appropriate facility being used? Is too much of a particular resource being used?

1991–today: The concept of health care value is now very complex, consisting of accessibility, necessity, utilization, quality, and satisfaction.

Information Systems

Information systems represent one of the most important factors in the design of the Business Architecture. Information systems can overcome physical obstacles and distances in the work flow; they can supply otherwise inaccessible data; they can assist in the performance of routine tasks; they can enforce policies; they can capture performance data; they can supplement the expertise of staff (medical expert systems); and they can assist in the development of new services.

This, of course, assumes that the hospital has assembled an effective Business Architecture. If it has poor or no controls, poorly designed activity flows, under-trained staff, or inappropriate organizational structures, then its attempts to automate the Business Architecture will be disappointments at best, and failures at worst.

MANAGEMENT DISCUSSION

Top management has little direct involvement with the Business Architecture. Nevertheless, it directly impacts the Business Architecture whenever it makes decisions about organizational structure, projects, or programs. Top management's feedback about the effectiveness of the hospital's Business processes comes from summary reports and external sources such as complaints and lawsuits; it does not deal directly with the processes. Management must understand the importance of its decisions on the value chain and communicate this downward. Top management cannot be expected to perform the analysis that would indicate the impact, but it should have an appreciation for the potential issues.

Understanding

Top management must adopt a "strategic" view of the Business processes. The "Seven S's" model (see Figure 4.7) is a powerful tool, popularized by McKinsey & Co., for assessing and communicating the "fit" among the components of the Business Architecture. The "S's" stand for Superordinate Goals, Strategy, Structure, Systems, Style, Staff, Skills. Their meanings are explained below:

Superordinate Goals: The mission, philosophy, and broad goals of the organization. Problems may arise when a new Strategy represents an unconscious departure from a hospital's prevailing Superordinate Goals. An example would be a not-for-profit hospital that adopts a financial strategy of creating a for-profit subsidiary to offset Medicaid/Medicare under-reimbursements. Is there still a fit between Superordinate Goals and Strategy? What other changes in organizational Structure or business Systems would be necessary to make this work? In many states, the attorneys general do not think there is a fit, and they are suing hospitals over this.

Strategy: The areas and ways in which the hospital will compete in

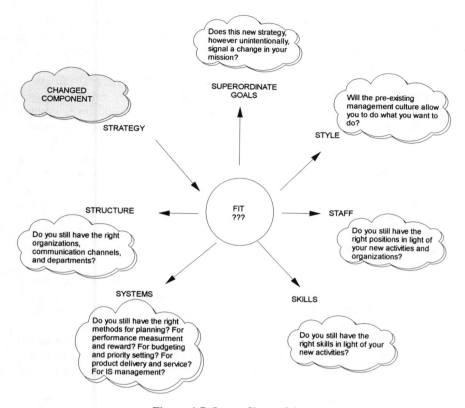

Figure 4.7 Seven S's model.

order to achieve its goals. This may also include information systems strategies. A strategy by itself may be appropriate, but the organizations and systems that are expected to carry it out may not fit with it. For example, the hospital might adopt a strategy of strengthening its relationships with physicians, using information systems. Unfortunately, the hospital gives the physicians access to a nonintegrated set of antiquated information systems, and provides no support to help them use the system.

Structure: The organizational structure of the hospital, including levels of authority and job descriptions. It also includes horizontal organizations such as committees and teams. Organizational structure includes issues like: is it a deep or flat hierarchy; is it a dual hierarchy (administration vs. medical staff); is it decentralized; is it a matrix? A Medical Records department with two directors (say, one for inpatient and one for out-patient) will impede efforts to implement a strategy of total quality. Another example: A decentralized hospital chain tries centralized support for information systems users. It establishes a centralized help desk, but does not have any support in the hospitals. In yet another case, the hospital desires to use information systems as a strategic tool, but keeps the VP of Information Systems under the CFO; this VP will never be allowed to develop the enterprise view of systems.

Systems: These are both business systems and information systems. A department can have one or more business systems. The process of chart management is a business system. The Pharmacy is a business system. Many systems have information system support. Some other, less obvious, systems would include, for example: how the hospital does budgeting, how the hospital prioritizes projects, and so forth. An example of poor use of systems would be when a hospital embarks on a new operation (e.g., home health) without looking at the related business processes: scheduling of staff, delivery of care, delivery of medical equipment and medicine, sending in charges and refilling inventory. Another example would be when a hospital commits thousands of dollars to establish a new program, such as a V.I.P registration card, but never defines the criteria for success.

Style: The management culture. Is management supportive or does it leave people to "fend for themselves"? Is it collegial or authoritarian? Is it insecure or self-confident? Is it "do as I do" or "do as I say"? Is failure tolerated? Is innovation encouraged? Is communication across departmental boundaries encouraged? Is disagreement valued and encouraged? If the strategy is to adopt an ongoing Total Quality Management (TQM) approach to hospital management, does a prevailing culture of punishment and defensiveness fit?

Staff: What are the job descriptions? Is there a chief technology officer? An MRI technician? If a strategic decision is made to pursue managed care, is there appropriate staffing for this (such as a managed care analyst)? If a strategic decision is made to make end users more self-sufficient, do the users have the right staff (such as a manager of departmental LANs)?

Skills: This is closely related to Staff. It encompasses the skills required by the staff in performance of their duties. This includes both technical and personal skills. Problems result when a hospital tries to staff a telemarketing operation with former billing staff without giving them the new skills; or when a hospital has an aggressive pricing campaign for a new operation, without any guidelines for staff when they consider discounting the service.

In all of this, there are very few absolutes. A conflict between staff and structure may be compensated temporarily by the charisma of an individual manager. But, in the long-run, this structural imbalance must be changed.

Whenever top management makes a decision about new programs, policies, or organizational structures it is in danger of upsetting the equilibrium of the Business Architecture.

Leadership

The material in this book will not be internalized without a hospital-wide shift in values and attitudes. Top management must encourage middle management to question their decisions in light of the Business Architecture, and middle management must do the same with supervisors and line personnel. This requires that management place its insecurities aside. Changes in attitudes do not occur without the active intervention of top management. This means that top management must descend into the details and "get dirty." Top management must understand what is at the end of its vision, and how to get there—the methods it will use.

The principles espoused by this book are consistent with those of TQM. People must be empowered: skills and culture play a role. Root causes must be corrected, not symptoms. The recent and quite legitimate growth in the use of total quality management is very encouraging for information systems professionals. This newfound interest in getting the business process right should carry over into information systems. It is interesting to note that, in the past, a request for an information system was frequently a tacit admission that a particular business process needed to be reengineered. However, rather than address the redesign of the Business Architecture directly, management relegated it to the information systems staff, making process redesign a result of systems implementation, rather than making systems implementation just one aspect of process redesign.

TECHNICAL DISCUSSION

No system—manual or automated—could be developed directly from the high-level diagram presented in Figure 4.8. The author actually saw a hospital consultant present this as an "architecture." Several levels and types of analysis are needed before a business process can be improved. The Business Architecture is literally a set of integrated blueprints of the hospital's business processes. Recall the discussion of the Seven S's model. A business process is one of the hospital's systems. From this point of view, Surgery is a business process; Admitting is a business process; ordering and preparing medications is a business process; and so forth. All of these processes are extremely complex—either techically or because of the need to interact with multiple departments. The reader should recall the architectural drawings for the construction of a new hospital wing. The drawings help the general manager assimilate the technical details. They also serve as documentation for what was agreed upon. Some of the drawings present the higher levels of detail, while others present the lower levels. This "leveling" is a response to a few basic realities:

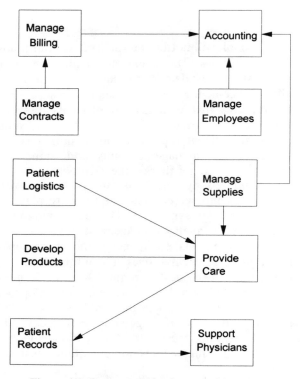

Figure 4.8 Purported "business architecture".

- An understanding of the logic behind a system must be achieved before one takes up the physical details.
- One cannot understand all the details at once.
- Organizations are composed of smaller units, but are part of a larger whole.
- Organizations are tied to each other in a multiplicity of ways: data flows, policies/procedures, technology, patient flows, and so on.
- Different organizations perform different types of activities.

Levels of Architecture

Figure 4.8 provides none of the detail needed to improve a hospital's business processes. It cannot answer any of the following questions:

- What types of staff and how many of each?
- What skills?

- What data?
- How does the work flow?
- What are the policies and procedures for each activity?
- What are the controls and measures of success?
- What is the relevance to strategy?
- What is the timing and sequencing of the activities?

This drawing is simply an abstract metaphor. It has value in that it serves to structure and focus a discussion, but it is definitely not an architecture. The challenge is to take the conceptual picture and provide additional levels of specificity in a way that moves closer to a physical implementation. No one can take the diagram from Figure 4.8 and turn it into an information system, with programs, files, hardware, staff, and controls. One cannot even begin to implement a business process without several levels of analysis.

Historically, there have been various approaches to the issue of business process engineering. They have been called different things: Systems Analysis, Industrial Engineering, and Management Engineering.

1. *Systems Analysis*: Concentrated on automating existing processes. It looked at the data flows among users in order to give them common access to data, but it did not look at the data of the enterprise. The logic of the process was studied only so that it could be automated. It did not link activities with objectives and measures; it was treated as a stand-alone activity, which did not need the support of higher levels of management.

2. *Industrial Engineering*: Concentrated on the efficient design of work flows and jobs; divorced from the total product; viewed by management as "beneath" their attention.

3. *Management Engineering*: Concentrated on examining job descriptions, measurements of performance; ignored total product picture; viewed by management as not worthy of their effort.

These approaches all had the same two flaws:

1. They were myopic, looking only at the job or the department. They missed the big picture. They did not consider the implications of the value chain (products and customers). They did not deal well with organizational interaction. They did not deal with organizational design.

2. They were performed within a management culture that did not appreciate the need for this activity and that did not promote the atmosphere needed for it to be successful.

The activity of business process engineering/reengineering can be done in either a reactive mode or a proactive mode. A TQM culture would dictate the latter.

Guidelines for Reengineering a Business Process

In light of what has been said, there are certain prerequisites for meaningful business reengineering: (1) It should be done by a team that crosses organizational boundaries, because business processes cross organizational boundaries; (2) it needs top management support, and this can be achieved only by getting top management to understand the process—management should attend training sessions to enhance this understanding; and (3) it requires the buy-in and participation of supervisors and line personnel. It also requires the right "culture," one that encourages people to think independently and to admit mistakes in a nonpunitive atmosphere. Culture represents a formidable obstacle in traditional hospitals, where doctors are viewed as infallible, departments are stand-alone, and administration is weak in leadership and technical skills. Meaningful business reengineering requires that all levels of hospital staff learn analytic disciplines and be proactive.[1]

The value chain can be viewed as a series of cycles: the Inbound Logistics cycle, the Product Operations cycle, and so forth. It is useful to break the value chain into cycles because this reinforces the idea that it is repeated, that it can be measured, and that there can be interactions among the phases within the cycle. In generic manufacturing, Inbound Logistics consists of ordering, receiving, storing, delivery, returns, and management control activities. Product Operations consists of design, manufacturing, assembly, testing, finishing, and management control activities. Health care also consists of a series of cycles. Its inbound logistics is similar to that of other industries. Product Operations includes the many product lines of the hospital (cardiology, surgery, general medicine).

These cycles consist of Phases. The phases can be broken down into activities. The activities can be broken down into tasks. (The different formal methodologies will have different names for these components.) This hierarchy is shown in Figure 4.9.

1. *Phase*: The stage through which the patient passes. For example, the major phases of a patient's stay in the hospital are the admitting phase, the assessment phase, the care provision phase, and the discharge phase.

---

[1] For a more radical approach to business process reengineering see Michael Hammer and James Champy, *Reengineering the Corporation: A Manifesto for Business Revolution*, New York: Harper Business, 1993.

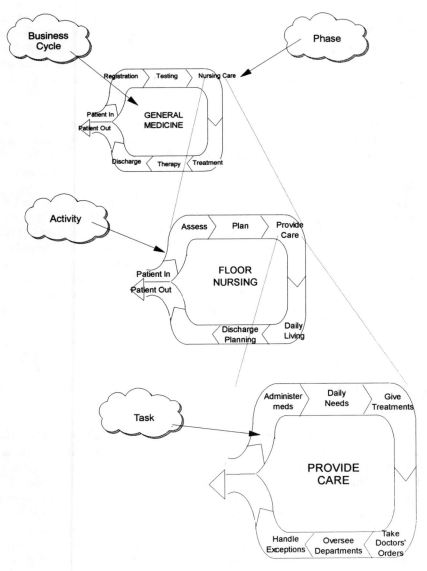

Figure 4.9 Hierarchy of cycles.

2. *Activity*: The activities of individual departments in support of a particular phase. For example, during the Nursing phase of a patient's hospital stay, Nursing performs the activities of administering medications, recording vital signs, family counseling, and so forth.

3. *Task*: These are the procedural aspects of the activity. As a rule, one can fix business processes only at this level, where a concrete person performs a concrete task(s). It is almost always necessary to provide this level of analysis to fix a problem. If one were going to design a department from scratch, one would have to do this. A task could be further analyzed into steps.

In addition to the activities directly associated with product development and delivery, there is a network of numerous support activities, which includes the traditional "ancillary" departments such as Lab and Pharmacy, as well as back-office activities such as accounting and marketing.

There is a distinction between the *logic* of a business process and its *physical structuring*. Figure 4.9 shows only the logic. As the analyst moves down to the task level he gets closer to the physical setup and flows of the business process. This can get "messy," and it is understandable only if the logic has been documented separately. In addition, you have to specify the organizations that execute and control this business process.

The guidelines for redesign are explained below. They include:

1. Define objectives

2. Document phases

3. Document activities

4. Document tasks

5. Redesign

The first two steps are for scoping; the second two are for analysis; the last step is for redesign. Keep in mind, however, that analysis is an iterative activity. While the analyst may have an idea of the general direction, he does not know what the final destination will look like. He will have to loop back, and be prepared to retrace his route. To illustrate this redesign method the text examines the redesign of certain aspects of nursing care. This is done in a context of *ongoing redesign* of an existing business process, which might be part of an ongoing TQM process. There is another type of design: *strategic redesign*, which will be discussed later in this chapter.

1. State the Departmental Objectives

When business processes are examined, it should be done in light of some strategy or business objectives. It is not enough to state, "Improve Nursing." It needs to be stated within the context of a strategy, such as, "Nursing will demonstrate consistently high levels in the quality of patient care, as measured by medication error rates, contributing to the hospital's strategy of winning over payers through recording and advertising its quality data." However, the scope needs to be narrowed. Is this all nursing departments, or just Floor Nursing? For the sake of argument, we will assume that the charge is to improve the quality of the care delivered on the Nursing floors. (Even though we start out with Nursing floors, we need to keep the big picture in mind.)

2. Analysis at the Phase Level

Document the generic business cycle and the supporting business cycles. This needs to be done in the context of the hospital's product lines. Each product line has a different cycle. A "cycle" is the set of activities or phases associated with the product as it is provided. Hospital product lines include general medical/surgical, transplants, dialysis, chemotherapy, psychiatry, pediatrics, and so forth. One also needs to look at who performs them, as well as the measures of success and the associated problems.

2.1 Draw the Cycle

This is for scoping and context. See Figure 4.10. The Registration phase includes any preregistration work, admitting, and bed assignment. The Testing phase includes initial testing, assessment, diagnosis, and planning. The Treatment phase includes clinical procedures, therapies, and nursing care. The Discharge phase includes discharge planning, filling out the medical record, and the actual discharge. This cycle is generic, and can be applied to all the product lines of the hospital, including outpatient services. A given product line will have its own distinctive set of supporting cycles, as shown in Figure 4.11. A cardiology patient will use

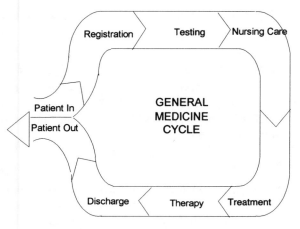

Figure 4.10 General medicine cycle.

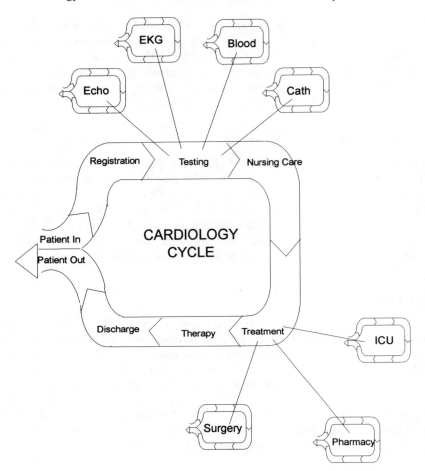

Figure 4.11 Cardiology and supporting cycles.

different services for the testing and assessment phases. This patient may also use surgical and ICU services. Many of these services can be performed in parallel, or a given service can be performed multiple times in succession (Lab, for example). At this level, one does not see the exceptions or the management activities.

2.2 Draw Ancillary Cycles

Draw the cycles for other business processes that both impact and are impacted by the business process under examination. The product-line cycles are oriented toward patient contact and patient flow. Each of them has one or more "ancillary" cycles, which include all their support

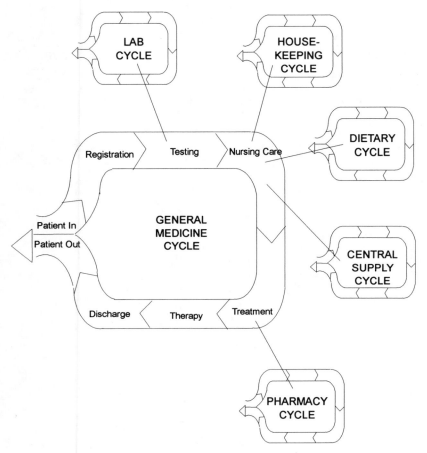

Figure 4.12 General medicine and supporting cycles.

organizations, not just the classical ancillary departments of pharmacy, radiology, and laboratory (see Figure 4.12).

This is done for scoping and analysis purposes. One fault of traditional systems analysis methodologies is that they treat entities outside of the local value chain as "black boxes." That is, analysis stops at the flow of data outside of the local department. Value-chain analysis requires that linkages be made between the local value chain and the value chains of other departments. One has to trace the impacts between the value chains. Impacts could include the following: communications, document transfer, doing something on someone's behalf. Note the cascade effect. The Nursing Unit is responsible for this phase and relies heavily on other departments for their support of nursing activities.

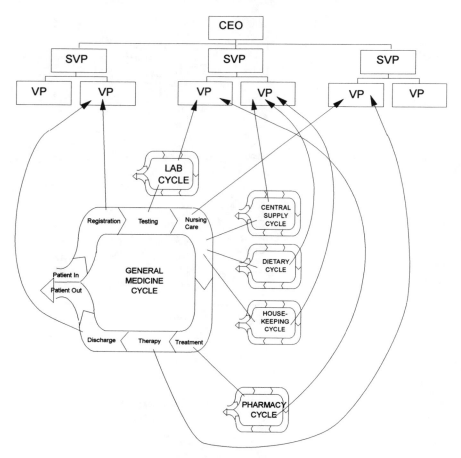

Figure 4.13 Cycles versus organizational structure.

2.3 Draw the Organizations

During any given phase, one particular organization will have primary responsibility for that phase, but relies on other organizations for services and data. For example, Nursing is responsible for the patients in the nursing units, but it also uses the services of Business Services, House-keeping, Medical Staff, Medical Records, Dietary, Pharmacy, and Lab. Problems occur when organizational borders interfere with communication, problem solving, and resource use. Figure 4.13 maps the cycles to the organizational chart of the hospital. It can be seen that the business process is controlled by six VPs who report to three different SVPs. The analyst needs to look for any organizational structures (teams, steering committees, etc.) that perform horizontal integration.

2.4 Draw the Cycle Problem Matrix

This is the last major item of analysis at the phase level. The diagrams developed previously permit the analyst to construct a matrix of the problems associated with these departmental interactions (see Table 4.1). This matrix matches the departments against each other. Those cells above the shaded area present the problems caused by Nursing *vis-à-vis other departments*. For example, Nursing creates a negative impact on the Lab when it mislabels specimens; it impacts Pharmacy when it does not update the medication records. The cells below the shaded area hold the problems that other departments cause *vis-à-vis Nursing*. For example, Pharmacy can provide the wrong dose for Nursing, which has to administer the medication.

This first matrix can be elaborated with a second matrix (Table 4.2) that provides more details about the impacts of these problems. The second matrix is labeled as "symptoms" because, at this early point, it is frequently impossible to assign a precise cause. Subsequent analysis will reveal the underlying causes and the ultimate impacts.

3. Analysis at the Activity Level

The analysis moves to the next level of detail—the activities that occur within each departmental cycle. For example, the Floor Nursing Care cycle consists of assessment, care plans, provision of care, help with daily living, and discharge planning. This is the level at which departmental problem solving occurs.

3.1 Record the Activities

The analyst must define the major activities at the activity level. This is done in Figure 4.14. Once again, an activity cycle is used to represent the business process. The nature of these activities can be quite different from one department to another. In Admitting, the activities are more sequential and less prone to random interruptions. On a nursing unit, however, the activities are less sequential, more parallel, and subject to frequent random interruptions. In Admitting, many transactions may be done in batches. Some activities are like an assembly line; others are like custom orders. Floor nursing is different from ICU nursing, where there is one nurse per patient. Lab may have an extended waiting period between the test and the result. So different techniques for analysis will have to be used.

This model is not meant to be completely sequential. The activities for each patient, or group of patients, do not necessarily occur in this sequence, and there is much random interruption and unplanned problem solving. Nevertheless, the model is valuable for conveying the fact that the purpose of the activities is to get the patient in and out efficiently and

Table 4.1 Cycle Problem Matrix—Simple

Impacting department	Impacted department							
	Nursing	Dietary	Pharmacy	Housekeeping	Medical Records	Laboratory	Central supply	Admitting
Nursing	Incorrect orders	Incorrect orders Updates to orders not communicated	Incorrect orders Updates to orders not communicated Mistakes in medication administration	Updates to orders not communicated Lack of priorities Unclear instruction	Misplaced Charts Delays in sending charts back at time of discharge	Mislabeling of specimens	Incorrect orders Updates to orders not communicated	Does not inform of discharge
Dietary	Wrong meals Wrong time							
Pharmacy	Wrong dose Wrong drug Wrong time Not available							
Housekeeping	Not there when needed Lack of supplies Wrong supplies Attitude Language							

Medical records — Nonavailabity of patient records

Laboratory — Not arriving when needed
Mislabeling of specimens
Lost specimens
Delays in getting results

Central supply — Wrong equipment
Shortages
Broken equipment
Delays

Admitting — Delays in providing info

Table 4.2 Cycle Problem Matrix—Expanded

Impacting department	Impacted department Nursing	
	Problems/symptoms	Impacts
Nursing	n/a	n/a
Dietary	Wrong meals Wrong time	Medications cannot be given when needed, impacting quality of care.
Pharmacy	Wrong dose Wrong drug Wrong time Not available	Wrong dose, wrong drug both impact quality of care and legal risks; wrong time is similar.
Housekeeping	Not there when needed Lack of supplies Wrong supplies Attitude Language	Patient and Nursing are inconvenienced, impacting costs and patient satisfaction.
Medical records	Volumes of paperwork Nonavailability of patient records	Data is not available when needed, impacting quality of care and legal risks.
Laboratory	Not arriving when needed Mislabeling of specimens Lost specimens Delays in getting results	Results are not available when needed, or the wrong result is provided, impacting patient care. Lost specimens cause delays, which increase costs, hurt patient satisfaction, and impact quality of care.
Central supply	Wrong equipment Shortages Broken equipment Delays	The resultant delays impact costs, patient satisfaction, and quality of care.
Admitting	Delays in providing info	Many intermediate impacts; Ultimately, the nursing staff has less time to spend on patient care, and a reduced ability to provide high-quality patient care.

to provide care while there. Other levels of analysis will show the flows. (This level is useful for planning the data base.)

3.2 Record the Measures

For each of the activities, document the theoretical measure of success. It should be quantifiable. Sometimes no measures are defined. Sometimes they are defined, but the actual measurement is not performed. In other cases, the measurement is performed, but no corrective action is taken. Some methodologies refer to this as "cycle time," but time is not the only measure. These measures represent the objectives of the activity.

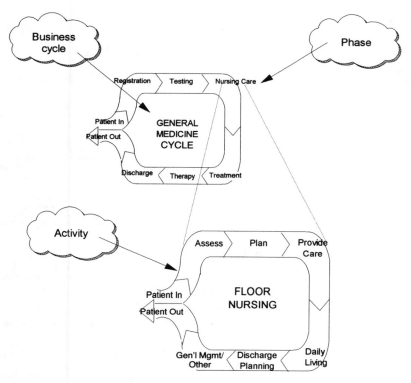

Figure 4.14 Business cycle decomposed into activity cycle.

3.3 Value-Chain Analysis

Next, develop a value-chain analysis for this set of activities. In cases where the measure is not being achieved, this analysis will help reveal the causes. Figure 4.15 presents a value chain, listing its "value detractors."

3.4 Record the Value-Chain Interactions

Examine the interactions between Nursing and the other departments (see Figure 4.16). You will recall that this was done previously, in Tables 4.1 and 4.2. However, these were at a higher level of detail. Sometimes it is sufficient to stay at a higher level of detail; at other times, you must go down a level.

In other methods of systems analysis these departments are considered "sinks," that is, recipients of data that are out of the scope of the project. In actuality, they are all participants in a phase called "residence on a floor." And thus, they are all candidates for redesign. They are connected

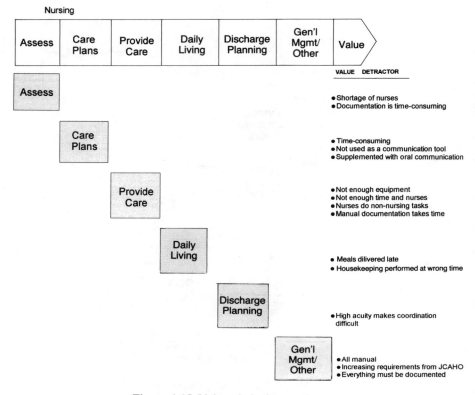

Figure 4.15 Value chain for nursing.

by common events. "Cleaning the room" is an event that requires the participation of several different departments.

3.5 Draw the Activity Problem Matrix

The matrix developed in Tables 4.1 and 4.2 is driven to a lower level of detail. For each activity in Figure 4.14, record the problems in a matrix format. As stated previously, many of these problems are really "symptoms." Table 4.3 matches each Nursing activity to the cycle of another department. Table 4.4 then documents the underlying causes for one of the Nursing activities—"Provide Care." It uses the Problems and Impacts from other tables and adds the Measures and Underlying Causes. A useful technique for getting at the underlying causes is to keep asking "why" until you arrive at the cause. At this level, there is frequently sufficient detail to discover the underlying causes of these problems. It is important to include Measures at this point. When the redesign occurs, it is greatly facilitated if there are objective criteria for determining the

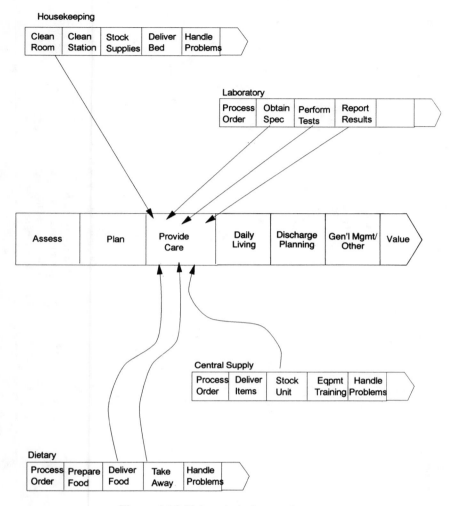

Figure 4.16 Value chain interactions.

successful performance of the activity. Moreover, the control activities must be built into the redesign of the process, and this allows for it.

4. Analysis at the Task Level

Next, the analyst must examine the value chain at the task level, identifying the data flows among the tasks. Each box should represent a procedure, and should be performed by a single person. Sometimes this level does not provide enough detail, and one or more activities must be further decomposed. For example, Provide Care is quite complex, consisting of administering medications, recording orders, and so on.

Table 4.3 Activity Problem Matrix—Simple

Impacting department	Impacted activity Nursing				
	Assess	Care plans	Provide care	Discharge planning	Document
Dietary	n/a	n/a	Meals not delivered on time	Dietician not available to assist with teaching	Tray taken away before intake can be documented
Pharmacy	n/a	n/a	n/a	Delays in getting meds for discharge, wrong volumes of meds	Stickers are missing or are not current
Housekeeping	n/a	n/a	Not there when needed, lack of supplies, wrong supplies	n/a	Items that need to be documented or assessed might be taken away by housekeeping staff
Medical records	Delays in obtaining the old records	n/a	Volumes of paperwork	n/a	n/a
Laboratory	Getting back initial lab work	n/a	Does not arrive when needed, mislabeling of specimens, lost specimens, delays in getting results	n/a	Obtaining results on time
Central supply	Getting supplies needed to admit and assess patient	n/a	Wrong equipment, shortages, broken equipment, delays	Difficult to obtain equipment for family to take home	n/a
Admitting	Delays in getting the initial paperwork	n/a	n/a	Difficult to clarify insurance coverage for take-home equipment	n/a

Table 4.4 Activity Problem Matrix—Expanded

Impacting department	Measure	Impacted nursing activity Provide care		
		Problem/ symptom	Impacts	Underlying causes
Dietary	The right meal delivered at the right time	See previous tables	See previous tables	Low-paying job
Pharmacy	The right medication delivered at the right time	See previous tables	See previous tables	Staffing, communications
Housekeeping	Both the unit and the rooms cleaned and stocked	See previous tables	See previous tables	Staffing, low pay, education, language
Medical records	Charts organized correctly and delivered on time	See previous tables	See previous tables	Staffing, system flows, hours, location
Laboratory	Specimens picked up and delivered on time, accurately labeled; results delivered on time	See previous tables	See previous tables	Staffing, system flows, hours, location
Central supply	Adequate levels of stock maintained, delivered on time and in working condition	See previous tables	See previous tables	Staffing levels, skills, language, system flows
Admitting	Data is complete and delivered on time	See previous tables	See previous tables	Staffing, system flows, hours, location

4.1 Identify the Tasks

Identify the tasks within each activity. Figure 4.17 displays a list of tasks for each activity within the Nursing cycle. There is a certain amount of trial and error in this analysis. As the analyst enumerates the tasks, he may find that some of them are sufficiently complex that they should be treated as separate activities. (Actually, such tasks could also be represented as a cycle, depending on their complexity.) Medication is an example.

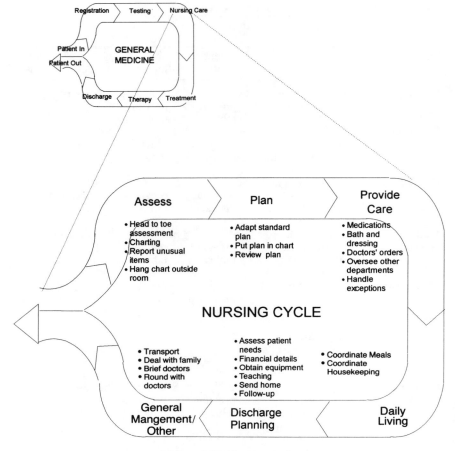

Figure 4.17 Nursing tasks.

4.2 Draw the Business Flows

Draw a flow diagram for each group of tasks. Figure 4.18 presents a dataflow diagram for Provide Care. The rounded rectangles represent the tasks. The text below the line in the rectangle indicates who performs this task. The shaded cycles represent related processes of other organizations. The open rectangles represent the storage of data. The labeled arrows represent the data that is used by this business process. This is where the diagrams show the physical structure of the business process, and where the work gets "messy." The stepwise decomposition of business processes takes the analyst from a more logical view to a more physical view. It is impossible to assimilate and manage these physical details without having a high-level context. End users from the business processes in question should be doing the analysis; however, when analyses get to this level of

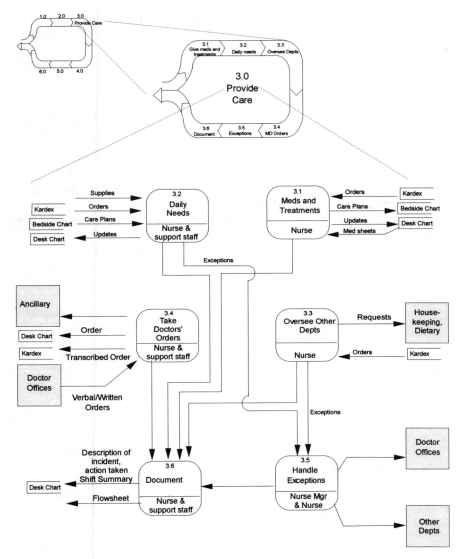

Figure 4.18 Flow diagram for nursing tasks.

detail, it can be useful to have a trained systems analyst assist with the dataflow diagrams, to help ensure consistency by observing the modeling conventions.

Sometimes it turns out that a given task is too complex and needs to be broken down into two or more tasks. This happens when a task is performed by more than one person, or is a decision node that branches into two or more tasks. Handle Exceptions is probably a decision node that branches into multiple tasks. Oversee Departments will have different kinds of outputs, which depend on different types of oversight tasks.

The six tasks shown in Figure 4.18 cannot be rigorously sequenced. They may proceed in parallel, with random interruptions. Tasks 3.1–3.5 are followed by a documentation task at the end of the shift, which was modeled separately since it occurs with a lag of several hours and since it contains the documentation of different tasks. (Obviously, many tasks have a simultaneous documentation step.)

There are many highly developed methodologies for systems analysis and design, each with its own conventions for representing activities and flows. This book does not claim to offer a full modeling methodology. This modeling technique is biased toward tasks, with other views secondary. There are other techniques for analyzing the flow of documents, the flow of materials, and the flow of patients and staff.

Regardless of the conventions, the methodology must ultimately permit the analyst to explicitly model the components of the business process at the task level, and these include data, procedures, controls, work flows, and staffing. These are defined in the next section.

One frequently finds numerous redundant steps, steps that need to be resequenced, or steps that should be performed by someone else.

These flow diagrams should be combined into a more comprehensive picture of the whole activity. This is done in Figure 4.19. Then these can be combined to show the flows for a whole phase.

4.3 Draw the Task Problem Matrix

Redraw the problem matrix for the task level of detail. This has been done in Table 4.5. At this low level, it is possible to provide a detailed classification of the problems by business process component. The major components are the following:

Organization: The hierarchical reporting relationships, horizontal coordinating teams, job responsibilities and authorities. This also includes culture and values.
Information: Data that is missing, late, or wrong. The classical reasons for automation.
Control (standards and measures): The performance standards; how they will be controlled.
Training (human resources): The number and types of staff, and their skill level.
Resources (other resources): Space, equipment, and so forth.
Work Flows: The flow of data, patients, staff, and materials and the spatial arrangement of the work areas.

At this level it should be possible to specify the root causes of problems. The flow diagrams show departmental connections, which allow greater

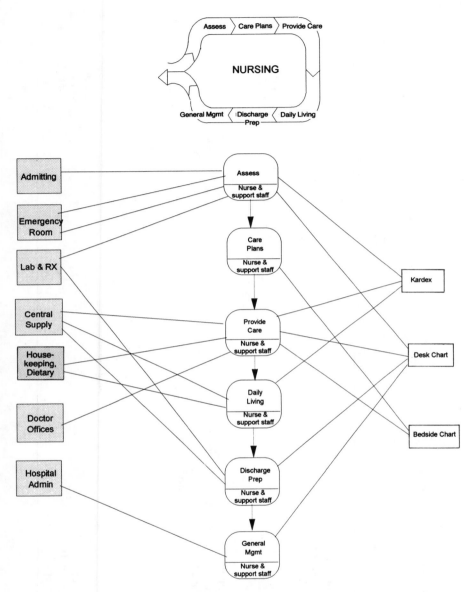

Figure 4.19 Consolidated flow diagram for nursing.

insight into "upstream" causes and "downstream" impacts. Different departments have different patterns of problems. Admitting might have problems with Information and Controls. A clinical research area might simply have Information problems. Nursing has Organization, Information, and Human Resource problems. Lab might have primarily Work Flow problems. Typically, problems occur in clusters. The most intract-

Table 4.5 Task Problem Matrix—Simple

Components of business processes	Breakdown of business activity Provide care					
	Administer meds	Daily needs	Give treatments	Take doctors' orders	Oversee other departments	Handle exceptions
Organizational structure	"Stovepipe" organizations, no teams				"Stovepipe" organizations, no teams	
Information availability	Order is not complete, nurse not familiar with medication			Order can't be read, is incomplete, or conflicts with other orders		Notes and communications get lost
Controls & measures	Shift-to-shift briefing is haphazard, no audits	"Complaints" and "outages" used as primary control mechanism			No jointly agreed-upon performance standards	
Training & skills						No training, in conflict management
Resources (facilities, equipment, $)			Management will not hire additional staff			
Flows	Many manual steps, redundant steps			Many manual steps, redundant steps		Many manual steps, redundant steps

able situation occurs when there is a management culture that is inimicable to fact-based analysis and team problem solving.

It is interesting that these root problem types resemble the Seven S's discussed earlier. This shows the connections between strategy and execution, and further reinforces the claim that if management adopts the right models, they will be equipped to deal with the lower levels of detail, and thus span the gulf between strategy and operations.

5. Redesign the Business Process

After the activities have been taken to the task level, the business process can be redesigned. Sometimes this redesign can span multiple processes and multiple departments. This frequently happens when the industry is undergoing rapid, fundamental change. In health care, some of the structural changes influencing redesign are: the switch to outpatient services; the growth of home health care; the new emphasis on the whole patient, including wellness and prevention; managed care; and the growing demand for quality measures.

The success of redesign depends on several factors. Within a single process or department, redesign is fairly staightforward. Business processes that span multiple departments, in which upstream activities impact downstream activities, can be very difficult to redesign. First, other managers may not share the interest in redesign, since it may cause certain functions to be eliminated, or may cause some functions to be moved from one department to another. This will be perceived as a threat. Second, the redesign may critically depend on the reliability of a new technology. In some cases, the technology may not be stable enough to support this redesign.

Redesign consists of one or more of the following structural changes, outlined in Table 4.6. They almost always occur in clusters.

1. *Policies and Procedures*: Policies may need to be redesigned to take into consideration the customer or other hospital departments. Staff may need to be educated concerning the policies. Policies may need to be enforced consistently.

2. *Skills and Training*: The lack of staff training is frequently a symptom of some other more fundamental problem. Hospitals hire staff at low wages, who have low skills. These people are thrown into action with minimal training. Correcting this problem requires a change in the management culture and value system.

3. *Restructuring of Work Flows*: This includes the elimination or reordering of tasks and the flow of information. Tasks may be reassigned to other organizations. Over the years, employees have come and gone, documentation has not been maintained, changes (manual and automated) have

Table 4.6 Task Problem Matrix—Expanded

Components of business processes	Breakdown of business activity Administer meds	
	Administer meds	Improvement opportunity
Organizational structure	"Stovepipe" organizations, no teams	Redesign care givers into teams and matrix organization, flatten existing structures, begin joint meetings.
Information availability	Order is not complete, nurse not familiar with medication	Have information system check for completeness, train and motivate nurses and physicians.
Controls & measures	Shift-to-shift briefing is haphazard, no audits	Establish a system for control.
Training & skills		
Resources (facilities, equipment, $)		
Flows	Many manual steps, redundant steps	Redesign flows, automating where possible.

been made to the business process. As a result, the procedural and flow aspects are confusing, and even incorrect. Most hospitals simply create incremental tasks and steps in response to new governmental and insurer requirements, rather than reanalyze the work flows.

4. *Redesign of the Organizational Hierarchy*: What was said about work flows also pertains to organizational structures. The organization charts of many hospitals reflect a historical period that long ago passed out of existence. While the industry has changed, moving from a monopoly to a free market service-oriented approach, the organizational design has not kept pace with changes in biomedical technology, information technology, and customer and payer demands. Hierarchical, vertical structures do not create flexible, responsive teams.

5. *Job Redesign*: The positions need their job descriptions updated to include performance standards and how they will be measured.

6. *Automated Support*: The volumes of data may be overwhelming the current manual process. However, before the process is automated, it should be redesigned. Most automation is used to support the traditional way of doing business. Even in those cases where it allows the hospital to work differently, it is force-fitted into the traditional manual environment. Example: A hospital acquires a patient accounting system that allows billers and collectors to communicate using electronic mail on-line. The hospital, however, continues to use handwritten notes and verbal communication.

7. *Measurement*: Whenever any change is made to the business process, the actual results must be compared with the previous results and the anticipated results. These are the measures of success. In some cases this requires sophisticated statistical analysis.

8. *Culture*: This is the ultimate redesign factor. All of the changes to components of the business process require the participation of humans. If the corporate culture does not encourage participation or fact-based, nonjudgmental analysis, then change will not be successful.

In many cases the diagrams and matrices that result from decomposing the business process are sufficient for analysis. There are other analysis and design techniques, however. Ishikawa ("fish bone") diagrams can be useful for associating cause and effect; methods of statistical process control can be useful for measuring results; management engineering techniques for defining productivity and quality standards are useful. Other types of diagrams, such as document flow diagrams and patient/material flow diagrams can contribute.[2]

5.1 Redesign the Organizational Structure

Frequently, the organizational structure is poorly aligned with the phases of the patient cycle, or with the tasks to be performed. Matrices can be helpful in showing these structural imbalances. This has been done in Table 4.7, which presents several activities and examines them for organizational effectiveness. It can be seen that they are not highly effective.

Beds: Nursing gets the immediate feedback from the patient and family; however, Nursing does not have the "upstream" responsibility. Housekeeping actually makes the bed. There is no common manager. There are no other organizational controls, such as review committees or teams, or task forces.

Table 4.7 Structural Imbalances in Cross-Departmental Activities

Activity	Organization	Immediate responsibility	Upstream responsibility	Common manager	Controls
Beds	Nursing	✓		No	
	Housekeeping		✓		Poor
Meals	Nursing	✓		No	
	Dietary		✓		Poor
Meds	Nursing	✓		No	
	Pharmacy		✓		Poor

---

[2] For a variety of analytic techniques, see Vincent K. Omachonn, *Total Quality and Productivity Management in Health Care Organizations*, Norcross; GA: Institute of Industrial Engineers, 1991.

Meals: The same situation. Nursing gets immediate feedback and evaluation, but they do not have the upstream responsibility. Dietary prepares and delivers the meals. Once again, there is no common manager; nor are there other organizational controls, such as review committees or teams.

Meds: Once again, Nursing gets the immediate feedback and evaluation, but does not have the upstream responsibility. Pharmacy prepares and delivers the meds. There is no common manager, and there are no other organizational controls.

It should be kept in mind that the reverse also holds. For many activities, Nursing is the upstream organization that causes problems for other downstream organizations. This happens, for example, when Nursing does not inform these organizations of changes in the patient's status.

Figure 4.20 makes this point graphically: How should the organization be changed to fit better with the business processes? There are different ways to approach the redesign. The hospital could simply train the employees better, including bringing them together for common training. Alternatively, the hospital could make structural changes, which could include (1) putting a single manager over both multiple functions (as a result, every department would report to Nursing); (2) creating teams that are responsible for the patient as he flows through the hospital; (3) creating a review committee.

A team leader could cut across organizational boundaries and get to the appropriate level of organization in order to resolve issues that arise with regard to coordination and communication. There probably would be different types of teams, depending on the diagnosis and services required by the patient.

In Figure 4.20 the same thing could be said about Admitting. They are the primary contact with patients during the Registration phase, but they depend on other organizations for critical inputs (insurers, Nursing, etc.).

5.2 Redesign the Business Process

Using what has been learned through matrix analysis, the hospital redesigns the business activities. This must be done at the task level. It has several aspects: procedural, human resources, controls, and automated tools.

Activities and Flows. A recent trend is to try to adopt the "best practices" within a particular industry. This practice is called "benchmarking." Hospitals with similar niches and size form peer groups and compare their practices across multiple business processes. A model practice is established, which hospitals then try to imitate. What hospitals need to realize, however, is that "culture" is also a best practice. Many best practices require that a management change its culture.

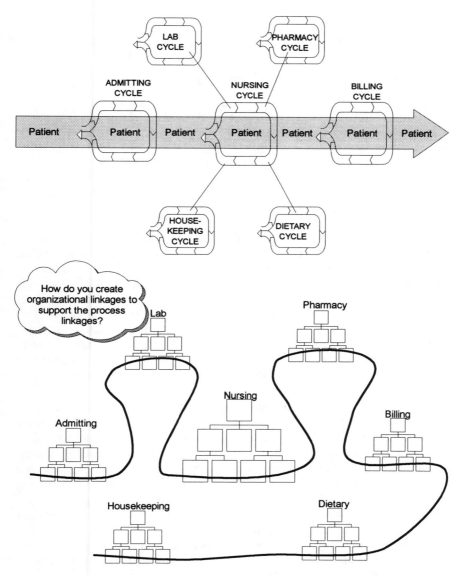

Figure 4.20 Patient flow linking activities and organizations.

Measures and Controls. There are different levels of measures (at the cycle level, the activity level, and the task level). Control has a business cycle of its own, which can be summarized as the "Four C's." They consist of Capturing the outcome, Comparing it to standards, Communicating it to the responsible person, and Correcting the problem and/or behavior. This generic control cycle is illustrated in Figure 4.21.

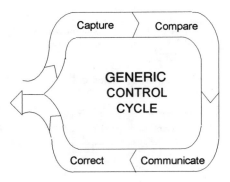

Figure 4.21 Generic control cycle.

This concentration on controls could easily lead to a bureaucratic night-mare. This is where computers play a critical role at each of these four control phases. It can be revealing to use the control cycle to examine the interactions between value chains. This is shown in Figure 4.22. Each side of the interaction (in this case, both the ordering and the delivery of meals) should have controls built into it. It is up to the hospital to determine how, when, and where it captures the data about the transaction; how, when, and where it compares the actual performance data to the standard; and so on. Figure 4.23 illustrates how a computer might be used to implement a control loop for the ordering of tests by a medical student.

Automated Tools. Information systems can prove useful, even critical, in the redesign of the business process. They are uniquely able to enforce consistency of policy and data, and to provide both fast recording of the data needed for quality, and fast follow-up and control. Unfortunately, in too many cases the information system is superimposed on a poorly designed manual process. Vendors have little interest in solving business problems. Hospitals have few skills and an improper mindset. And there are few tools to help with this. Requests for proposals are not developed to elucidate architecture.

After the hospital establishes its business architecture and systems architecture, it matches these to vendor alternatives. This match occurs at several levels. At the cycle level, the proposed information system must fit the hospital's business systems architecture. For example, we can see that a single patient is flowing across multiple departments (see Figure 4.20), but the data bases may be structured as stand-alone, so that Admitting has its version of the patient, Lab has its version of the patient, and Nursing has its own version of the patient. This will be addressed in Chapter 5: Data Architecture. In similar fashion, each department may have its own network to support patient care, and so the information systems "fragment" the business process.

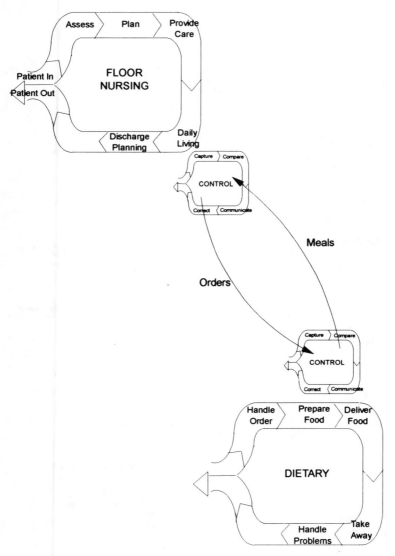

Figure 4.22 Controls on both sides of value chain interaction.

At the task level, does the proposed system do the required things: preregister a patient; create a demand bill; combine Lab and Pharmacy data? Does it do the right things in the right sequence: put a patient in the data base without creating an account; record a tentative outpatient visit without creating an account; create a charge only after the service is rendered; create a charge when the service is ordered; decrement inventory before it is picked/after it is picked? Does the system support

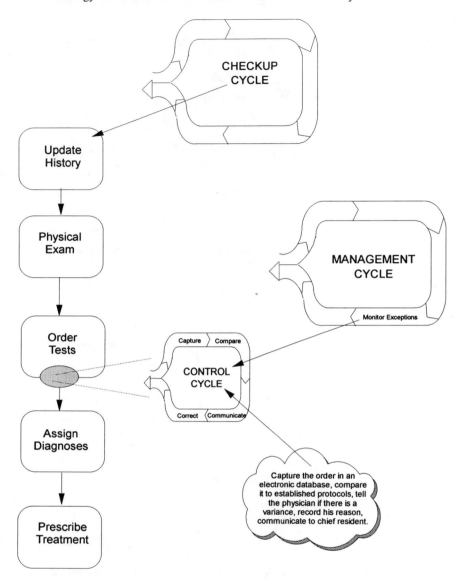

Figure 4.23 Control cycle for ordering of tests.

the data: multiple attending physicians per stay; accounts for other institutions, not just for individual patients?

At the task level, the analysis is mapped into screens, reports, and input documents. Does the system support the logic of each business task, such as determining financial class? Then there are the performance requirements: The hospital must analyze its business transactions for their

Table 4.8 Actual vs. Ideal RFP

Actual RFP process	Ideal RFP process
Discover "symptoms"	Discover "symptoms"
Write RFP	Discover "causes"
Acquire information system	Write RFP
Discover "causes"	Adjust information system to process
Adjust process to information system	Acquire information system

type, size, frequency, and their demands on system availability. Where do printers need to be located; are there any environmental issues such as emergency power, air conditioning, and security? Then one has to see whether the new system can accommodate this traffic.

In some cases, a new technology will force the hospital to restructure its business processes. For example, the introduction of an ICU information system that allows the monitoring of each patient from a single remote location has profound implications for scheduling and job design. Similarly, an electronic medical record system, or a type of imaging system, can introduce significant change into the business process. This is further exacerbated by the fact that microprocessors are being embedded in most medical devices. This provides greater control and features. It also provides the possibility for data management through these devices.

Request for Proposal. The addition of microprocessors has implications for the RFP process. The term "RFP" stands for Request for Proposal, a vehicle that specifies the requirements for an information system. The problem with almost every RFP is that it deals with symptoms and does not address the underlying causes of the problems and the redesign of the business process. Consequently, the reengineering is done as an afterthought, after the software has already been purchased. The RFP process itself is simply another of the hospital's business processes, which deserves to be redesigned. See Table 4.8.

New Business Processes

The preceding sections have shown techniques for redesigning existing business processes in the context of existing strategies. The same techniques can be applied to the design of new activities required by the introduction of new products or programs. For example, a hospital in the course of its strategic planning may decide that several major trends point to the need to actively pursue managed care. In the past, the hospital had accepted managed care patients, but on a limited scale and with a relatively small discount. Now, however, the hospital desires to integrate managed care principles into its philosophy and operations.

Top management assembles functional managers and department heads to assign projects that will produce the infrastructure for executing this new strategy. Marketing develops a marketing plan and advertising materials. Finance develops prices and costs. The Medical Staff department develops recruiting materials. Information systems look at data base issues. However, in all of this, the hospital assumes that existing departments may simply be extended in terms of functions and staff for this new activity. Coordination is performed by a project leader, and there are joint meetings. But the orientation is all bottom up. The resulting business process design is very department-oriented and likely not to look very different from the current operation.

Strategic Redesign Approach

This approach starts with strategy and a "clean slate." This approach is used in one of two ways: (1) to explicitly design the business processes that implement a *new* strategy; or (2) to redesign existing processes in a company that has lagged behind the overall rate of change in an industry, and which desires to achieve more than incremental improvement—it desires quantum improvement. In both cases, it starts with a clean slate, as much as possible unbiased by existing processes and purported "constraints." It is driven by a vision of how things "could" or "should" be, reinforced by the reality of objectives and measures. After this ideal design is achieved, it is mapped to specific organizations and business flows. This design activity can benefit from the use of consultants, who are able to avoid traditional biases within the company.

Strategic redesign has four major steps:

1. Identify structural characteristics of the industry.

2. Define strategy and vision.

3. Link strategy and vision to business processes.

4. Design processes based on strategy.

1. Identify Structure of Industry

A strong understanding of industry structure and trends should inform the hospital vision. While the strategic vision should not be limited by existing constraints such as organizational hierarchies and business flows, it should be conditioned by competitive realities such as competitor strength, market size, power of consolidated customers, and so forth. Figure 4.24 graphically illustrates the structural changes in the health care industry. The structural foundations of the industry—third-party payments with little control over the consumer of the services, intervention, and the independence of physicians—are shifting.

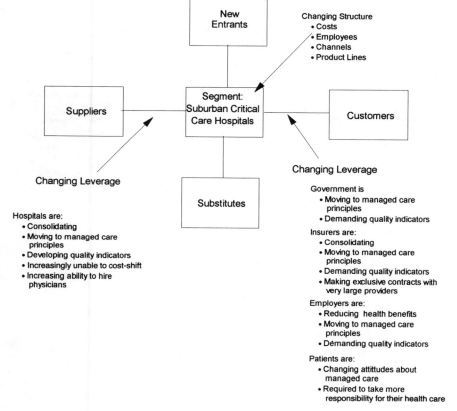

Figure 4.24 Changes in the health care industry.

2. Define Strategy and Vision

Management develops a new strategy set, specifying the need to build closer ties to large employers and insurers, to avoid duplication through consolidation, and to adopt managed care principles of operation. Management then goes on to brainstorm the ideal business cycles and business processes. This is shown in Figure 4.25, which represents a new vision of the world. It is no longer hospital-centric and hierarchical. It is focused on the customer and the product. An important aspect of managed care is that the care provider views the patient's condition as a continuum. At this level, management begins to specify the characteristics of the process and the measures of success.

3. Link Strategy and Vision to Processes

Design is moved down to lower levels. It is necessary to augment the team of senior managers with staff from lower levels to do this task. They

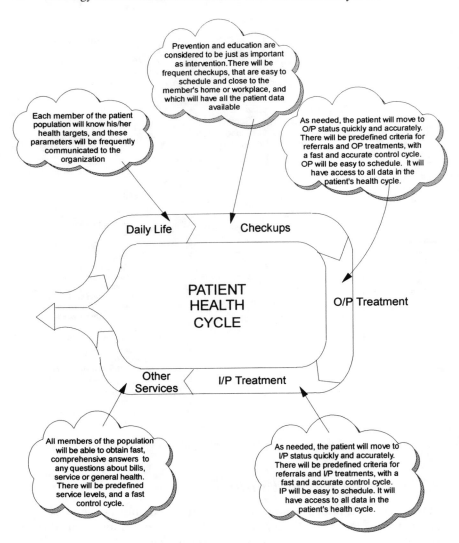

Figure 4.25 Ideal cycle for patients.

should brainstorm the most important objectives and characteristics of the new business processes. The five highest ranked characteristics might turn out to be:

1. Attracting managed-care business by recording and sharing performance indicators with insurers and payers.

2. Keeping costs down (by controlling resource use, using the most efficient resources, and by looking for economies of scale).

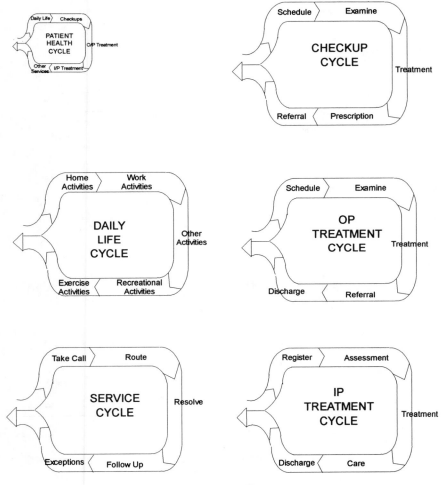

Figure 4.26 Cycles within patient health cycle.

3. Projecting demand accurately by understanding the patient population.

4. Designing clinical operations that match the demands of managed care principles.

5. Recruiting and retaining staff to perform managed care.

As the processes are redesigned, these factors are kept in mind. Figure 4.26 contains the next layer of detail, showing the subcycles within the Patient Health cycle. A management vision needs to be defined for each of these subcycles. The framework for this has been provided in Figure 4.27 for the IP Treatment cycle. This vision consists of the critical success

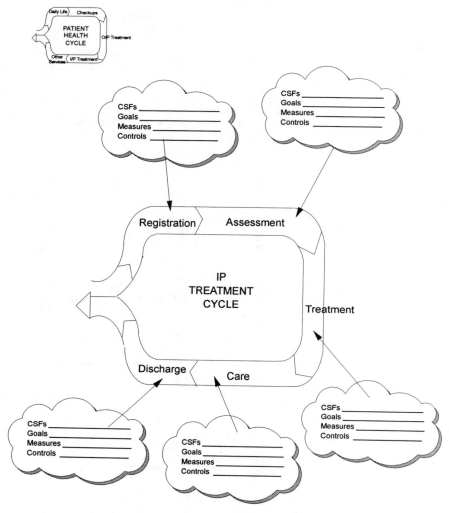

Figure 4.27 Framework for defining a vision of the inpatient treatment cycle.

factors, goals, measures, and controls, but leaves the physical details undefined. These characteristics would be defined for each of the activities within the cycle. They are further refined at the next lower level, as shown in Figure 4.28.

4. Design at the Process Level

Eventually, the design will be driven to the task and flow level, culminating in the specifications of the major components of the business process:

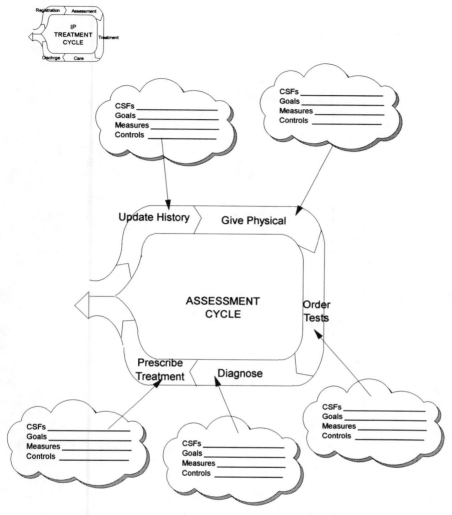

Figure 4.28 Framework for defining a vision of the assessment cycle.

staff, flows, procedures, controls, measures, information, organization. This process is somewhat different from the matrix-based top-down analysis done with the traditional approach to process re/design. Instead, the strategy drives an operational vision, and this vision is pushed down to the flow diagrams of the business process. At the level of the flows, each component is defined for the ideal system. In this process, emphasis is on the business process, without regard to existing organizational boundaries, staff skills, or information systems.

Table 4.9 Feasibility of Managed Care

Components of business processes	Breakdown of business activity Managed care				
	Attract business	Project demand	Control costs	Provide care	Recruit & retain staff
Organizational structure	Few linkages with primary care physicians and clinics			"Stovepipe" organizations prevent coordination needed for managed care	Hospital does not have sufficient in-house physicians for managed care
Information availability	Hospital info systems do not have ability to track and distribute data on costs, quality, and satisfaction	Information systems cannot support this	Information systems cannot track costs		
Controls & measures			Few cost controls are in place	Hospital has no controls in place for a managed care environment	

Training & skills	No one in hospital has skills and/or experience in marketing managed care on a wide scale	No one on staff has experience with projecting demand	Current staff is trained according to an "interventionist" model
Resources (facilities, equipment, $)		Current facilities are not cost-effective for the running of a managed care operation	
Flows			Current patient and staff flows do not support managed care

After one has gotten to the level of the "ideal" activities, one could use matrix analysis to understand more clearly what changes have to be made to existing components. This has been done in Table 4.9, which examines feasibility in light of critical success factors. These matrices could be applied to the task level as well.

5
Data Architecture

GENERAL DISCUSSION

The correct business processes and organizational structure are necessary, but they are not sufficient. Just as the organization and its processes must be structured correctly, so the data must also be structured correctly. This structuring is the Data Architecture. Staff need data in the performance of their duties. Having the right data available at the right time allows the hospital to provide better service. It tightens the control cycles, smoothes transitions, and adds value to services by embedding information in them. The data must be structured both logically and physically. That is, one must know the definition of a Patient, and one must know how to relate the Patient data in the Registration files with the Patient data in the Laboratory system.

The rather simple model in Figure 5.1 states that the hospital needs to maintain a "big picture" view of patients as they pass from one phase (or department) to another. Each department has its own specialized view of the patient. However, an enterprise view is needed to ensure end-to-end quality. This enterprise view requires that the hospital access and manipulate the patient as an entity separate from the visit.

If the data is not available at certain key junctures, or if it is incorrect or incomplete, it produces "service discontinuities." If it is structured wrong, this can prevent the hospital from operating as it desires. Service discontinuities are particularly noticeable when a hospital employs multiple information systems; however, the same thing can happen in a manual process. These critical junctures can be seen in the Business Architecture. The term "system interface," while originally used to describe the passing of data from one computer to another, can also be used to describe the departmental interactions that occur during a patient

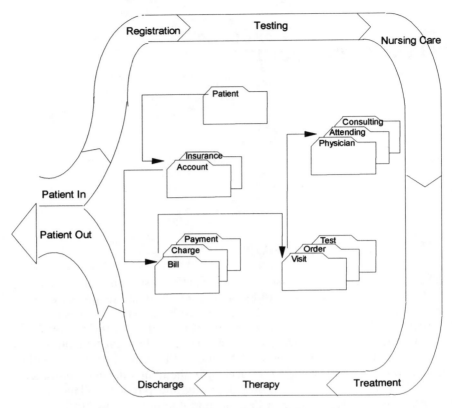

Figure 5.1 "Big Picture" view of the patient.

encounter. Figure 5.2 shows the interaction among several value chains, with the Nursing cycle as its focus. At every point of interaction there is the risk of losing or distorting data, whether the interaction is manual or automated. That is, it reduces the "value-added" of the activity. Figure 5.3 shows the value detractors for Nursing. Many of them are data related.

Industry Change and Data

When an industry undergoes fundamental structural change, the data underlying a company's business model also changes. Chapter 2 discussed the structural characteristics of industries, and how they can be altered by changes in the environment or by the initiatives of individual competitors. The environmental factors include politics, economics, demographics, social trends, and so forth. The resulting structural changes include the following:

- Providers become more consolidated.
- The influence of payers may shift.
- Channels for health care delivery change (e.g., the shift to out-patient care, same-day surgery, and home health care).
- The nature and amount of inputs change, and cause cost structures to change.
- Government regulations, requiring the reporting of new types of data or newly correlated data, may change.

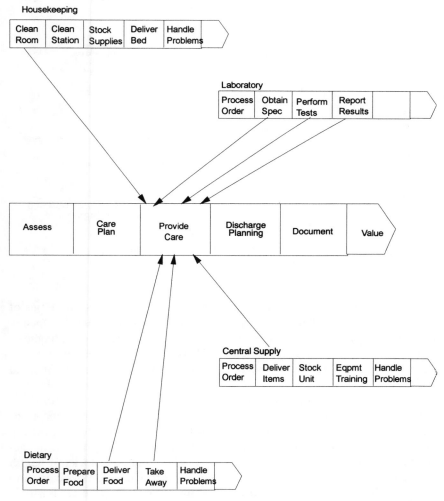

Figure 5.2 Value chain interactions.

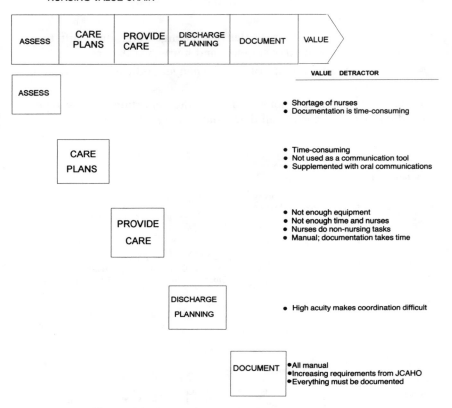

Figure 5.3 Value detractors in nursing value chain.

As the industry changes, it causes changes in the amounts and types of data that must be collected and managed. This data is needed (1) to stay in business (regulatory); (2) to provide better care and service (outcomes); or (3) to manage resources more efficiently (costs). These are not mutually exclusive. Table 5.1 lists some of the more important changes in data collection.

The architectural metaphor adopted by this book is quite appropriate, because computerized data is physically stored in blocks, with connections among these blocks. The arrangement of these blocks should support the hospital's business model, to facilitate management and reporting according to a particular model of the world. The building blocks of health care data are Patient, Diagnosis, Procedure, Bill, Charge, Physician, and so forth. The top half of Figure 5.4 shows a simple hospital business model. Its logic is the following:

Table 5.1 Increasing Data Requirements for Hospitals

Industry phase	Added requirements for data collection
1945–1965 Gov't-sponsored growth; supply emphasized; other aspects of industry remain relatively traditional.	• Patient demographics • Insurance
1965–1973 Medicare/Medicaid introduced; access now emphasized; Government paid—privately provided. Significant groups not included (poor, children). Health care becomes a big business.	• Medicare data • Medicaid data
1973–1983 Costs grow; disenchantment on many fronts; U.S. loses some competitiveness, goes off gold standard; For-profit hospitals emerge. Chains emerge. CON introduced.	• Extra insurance data • Coverage data • UB-82 data • Utilization data • Marketing data
1983–1991 Disenchantment grows. DRGs introduced. Emphasis on cost (then quality). Hospital profits decrease dramatically, but costs grow.	• DRG data • Cost data • Quality data • Risk data • Authorization data
1991– Universal dissatisfaction; National practitioner data base; All constituents agree that health care must be changed fundamentally; more systemic view of problems; threat of greater gov't involvement; combined emphasis on cost + quality + satisfaction.	• Government intends to require significant additional data related to outcomes. • Health care reform, no matter what form it takes, will require massive additional data collection.

A physician admits the patient and assigns a diagnosis. He orders services and also provides some of them. The patient receives an account. Services are charged to accounts and listed in bills.

Over time, however, the structure of the world (i.e., a particular industry and its environment) changes, necessitating changes to the data building blocks: new building blocks appear (insurance verification); new connections are created among existing blocks (between Diagnosis and Procedure). This concept is illustrated in the bottom half of Figure 5.4. Regulation causes the introduction of a new type of data called DRG. Competition causes hospitals to consolidate into chains, introducing a type of data called Facility. Payers begin to require that hospitals obtain authorization before they admit a patient, so Authorization data begins

Old

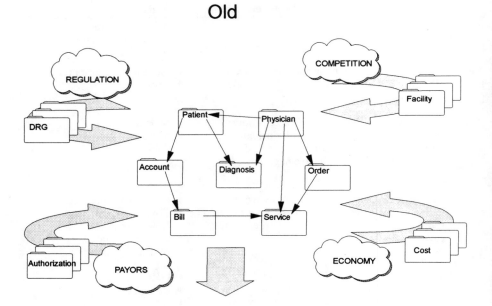

New

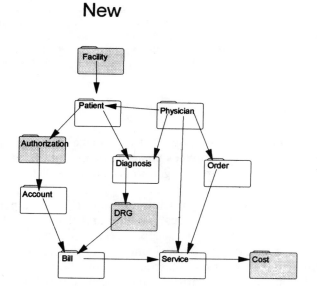

Figure 5.4 Old model of hospital logic, change factors, and new model.

to be collected. The economy changes (reinforced by political factors), causing hospitals to track Cost data. The logic of the business thus changes:

> When the patient is being admitted, the hospital must obtain an authorization from the payer. When a service is created, its costs must be estimated. When a patient is admitted, he must be associated with a specific facility. When a diagnosis is being assigned and the bill is being calculated, the DRG must be determined.

System Rigidity

Vendors develop information systems for an industry at a particular point in time. The data, together with the programs for storing, distributing, and processing it, reflect the specific business needs of the age, within the constraints of the available technology. When the industry changes, it is not a trivial task for the vendor to upgrade his product: The data must be restructured; the programs must be rewritten; screens and reports must be redesigned. Technology is both complex and rigid. System inflexibility is not a liability, as long as the industry is stable. Health care has undergone fundamental structural change in the past ten years, yet the structure of many hospital information systems reflects a fifteen-year-old data design.

Some systems still do not have a real patient Master File, separate from the visits (or accounts). Instead, if the hospital wants to look up a Patient, it must access the Visits. This makes it difficult to understand the hospital's customer base or provide prompt service to both patient and payer; it also makes it easier to issue duplicate medical record numbers. Some vendors have their Inpatient Registration system separate from the Outpatient Registration system; the two do not interact to provide an integrated view of the "Patient." In the 1970s, when the systems were designed, there were good reasons for this:

- Technology made integration difficult.
- Regulators did not require it.
- Competitive reasons did not require it. There was no concept of service. Hospitals were making money.
- DRGs had not yet been introduced, and there was little utilization review.

A recent ominous trend for hospitals is the formation of consortiums by the largest employers within a city, in order to share data about the city's health care providers. These consortiums are creating data bases that have quality, satisfaction, and cost indicators for each hospital's services. Consortium members compare hospitals to determine which appears to have the best mix of these indicators. Insurers are building the same types of data bases. The implications for hospitals are far-reaching. If hospitals do not restructure their own systems to measure and report such data, they will be at a disadvantage in negotiations.

A Data Architecture permits a hospital to match the data in its computer systems to its current business model at a particular point in an industry; when the industry starts to change, the model then allows the hospital to restructure its data assets to support new strategies and business processes.

Since the beginning of hospital information systems, and continuing today, vendors have been developing systems without an explicit data model. Consequently, the business model underlying the vendors' systems was not really the appropriate one. Systems from two different vendors were not readily comparable—in many cases they were both logically and physically incompatible. The definition of "outpatient" or "late charge" or "bill" was different from one system to another. Or, when it became necessary to extend the data base to accommodate costs and product lines, the data bases proved unintelligible and incompatible.

Data Management

Recall the "Technology/Methodology Lag" model presented in Chapter 2. When a technology is introduced, five to ten years pass before industries develop effective methodologies for its use. There have been several generations of data base management software, but advances in data management techniques have been slow. Mainframe data base management systems were introduced in the early 1970s; methodologies to exploit this technology began to appear in the early 1980s. In the early 1980s PC and LAN data base management systems appeared; there are still relatively few instances of their effective use to integrate departments, to say nothing of the enterprise. The next generation of DBMSs (distributed data base management systems) will store and retrieve data across multiple networks and hardware platforms. This technology will permit management of all data across an enterprise, presenting heretofore unimagined possibilities for aligning data with business processes. However, effective methods for analysis, design, and control do not exist, and will probably not appear until the late 1990s.

Traditional Methods and Tools

Traditional systems analysis and design is based on a "process" view of the world, as illustrated by the flow chart in Figure 5.5. In this view, a business process occurs, runs to completion, and then passes data to the

BUSINESS PROCESS

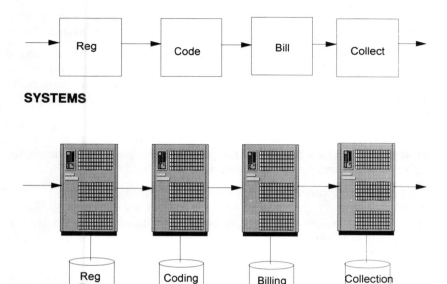

Figure 5.5 "Process" view of the world.

next business process down the line. And in reality, many business processes do indeed exhibit a serial behavior: The hospital must determine a patient's financial status before it sets up an account; an account must be set up before any charging can be done; diagnoses must be coded before they can be billed. The situation is similar for the clinical side of the hospital: An account must be set up before an order can be written; orders must be approved by a physician before they can be filled; results must be reviewed before they are released; and so forth.

Traditional information systems reflect this "serial" view of the world by setting up a series of files: File #1 is used as input to file #2; file #2 is used as input to file #3, and so on. This design results from the uninformed observation that each department had its own files before automation; it received data, kept its own copy, and then passed it on. Thus one can find a file for each department post-automation.

In reality, the reason departments keep their own copies of the data is that a manual filing system does not permit simultaneous access to a single file by many people from many locations. And so the analytic model is wrong. If one generalist person performed all the functions, there would be no data flows or multiple copies of data. The price of departmental specialization is the sequential flows of data from one department to another, with its attendant redundancy and inconsistency.

This serial design ignores the two-way interactions between value chains, and thus creates a series of operational problems. The systems, which are meant to support the business, do not follow its business logic:

1. Hospital staff often find that patient demographic data has changed when they are doing billing, scheduling, and collecting. Do you update the system you are working in and then send the data to the registration system? If you update the registration system, will the update get passed on to the billing system?

2. The price of a test is changed in the lab system on day x. On that same day, the person scheduling the patient's visit quotes the price in the registration system, which will be updated only on day x+2.

3. The bill is recorded as "paid" by the accounting system on day x, but the registration system does not know about it until day x+1. In the meantime, the patient waiting to be admitted is inconvenienced until this discrepancy is resolved.

While this serial design can be found even in single-vendor solutions, the problem is greatly exacerbated when a hospital employs applications from multiple HIS vendors.

Traditional methods for developing information systems emphasized automating the manual processes of an organization. The focus was on the activities, and data was secondary. Data was treated as the "by-product" of automation, without a value of its own. Historically, there are several valid explanations for the process-oriented approach:

1. *Perceived Need*: The first nonclinical activities to be automated had relatively low prestige and had clear efficiency motivation. (It is interesting to note that, on the clinical side, the value of the information was always appreciated by the practitioners.)

2. *Technology*: For nearly twenty years, the technology did not allow for on-line access to an integrated pool of data. The required progress in data management and telecommunications have occurred only in the past ten years. Initially, there were no interactive programs, and jobs were run in batches. The first storage medium was punched cards. Then came tape. This was followed by on-line storage of files. However, these files were stand-alone, and did not have data management programs to synchronize them. Finally, data base management software arrived on the scene.

3. *Methodology*: The methodologies were developed in the late 1970s, but were very slow to gain acceptance. Obviously, a data-oriented approach requires a new world view, like the shift from geocentrism to heliocentrism. It also requires new business processes and new manage-

ment controls (see Chapter 7: Control Architecture). All this took a long time to evolve.

4. *Tools*: The methodologies were hindered by practical considerations. The methodologies require that a huge number of data elements be defined. This then has to be maintained. Finally, it needs to be integrated with the systems development and configuration management processes. All of this requires the use of tools such as graphics, integrated with word processing and data base software, data modeling software, data dictionary software, CASE software. Most of these tools became widely available only in the late 1980s. (Furthermore, there is a methodological lag in learning how to use the tools effectively.)

The design implications were the following: Information systems usually exchange data in batch interfaces overnight, if they exchange data at all. This design imposes unnatural organizational boundaries. It would be unthinkable for a hospital to declare that the registration department could not call the scheduling staff, and vice versa. But this is precisely the artificial boundary that systems have produced. In simpler times, or in simpler hospitals where there is a manual system, either the same staff perform multiple functions, or they pick up the phone or walk over to their colleagues and obtain the information that they need.

New Approaches to Data Management

Starting with the 1980s, alternative methods for data management were introduced. This is the "data-driven" approach, and it represented a radical change in perception and methods. With regard to perception, it required that the hospital stop thinking that systems and data bases "flow" one into another. On the contrary, all systems are part of a common data resource. Individual systems merely collect and distribute this common data, as well as perform special processing and formatting. Regardless of the diversity among departmental activities, the data is common to all areas. With regard to methods, the data-driven approach requires that the hospital build a model of the data that underlies the process to be automated, instead of mechanically automating the visible data flows. When the hospital develops an information system, it should not assume that it has stand-alone logic. The hospital must determine how the system relates to the overall hospital data model, and how it can be synchronized with the other systems in light of that model.

The patient care process, while it does have serial aspects, also shows parallel and iterative activities. A physician can interrupt what he is doing to inquire about the status of X-rays; he may loop back to examine the details of a previous visit; or he may reorder a test. A given department needs to know what is going on simultaneously in another department: A surgeon needs to know what is going in Pathology; a registration clerk needs to know what is going on in the billing department; and so on. Traditional serial design is unable to capture the phases through which a patient passes. A patient goes through many states with regard to a hospital stay (or a clinic visit). The patient is recorded as a patient, gets an account, gets registered for an encounter, gets treated, gets discharged, and gets billed. There may be multiple departments, but there is a single patient. There may be multiple physical data bases, but they interact in such a way that they preserve the underlying logic of the data. And so a simultaneous, global approach to the data is needed. This situation is illustrated in Figure 5.6. Traditional serial design also emphasizes the horizontal dimension of data—its flow through a single episode. It often ignores the vertical dimension—data retention.

Other industries adopted the data-driven approach sooner than health care. But by the late 1980s and early 1990s one can find pockets of expertise and practice. They are motivated by the competitive environment and aided by advances in technology, including LANs; relational data bases; data bases that run on many different hardware platforms; SQL, which allows data access across multiple systems; and tools for drawing and maintaining models of hospital data. More recently, the philosophy and methods of TQM and business process reengineering have confirmed the validity of the data-driven approach.

Historical Summary

Table 5.2 summarizes the trends by historical era.

1960s: Information technology is new. There is no technology and no methods for data management. Data is locked in centralized files.

1970s: For the first time, technology allows the initial steps toward data management. Minicomputers can hold data locally. On-line disk drives and CRTs simplify data access. Mainframe data base management systems are introduced, more as a way to simplify file management than to manage data across a company. Structured analysis and design methods are a way to understand data flows produced by processes and to structure master files.

1980s: PCs are introduced, allowing data management at the desktop. This gives rise to PC DBMS's. The relational approach is used, because previous models of data bases are too complex for end users to understand. The data-driven view of the world challenges the process view. In order to understand how the company's data fits together, the Data Administration function is started, distinct from the Data Base Administration function, which concentrated on the performance, security, and backup of data bases.

1990s: PCs acquire the features of mainframes: redundant components, high-speed disks, backup power, and so on. They are now ready to apply mainframe techniques at the local level. Enterprise networks allow dis-

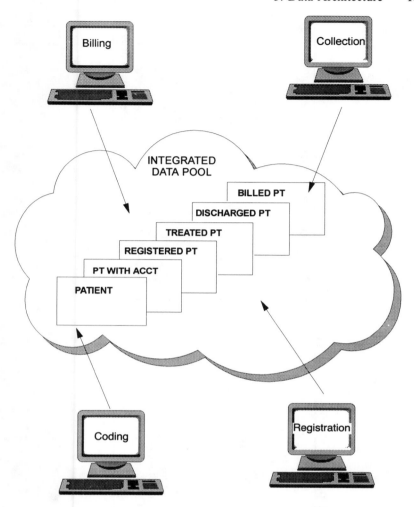

Figure 5.6 "Data-driven" view of the world.

tribution of data across the company. As networks become capable of carrying multiple data types simultaneously (moving images, wave forms, voice, handwriting, unstructured text), object modeling challenges relational modeling.

MANAGEMENT DISCUSSION

Top management's exposure to data architecture is the frustration it experiences when it discovers that the logic of the information systems

Table 5.2 Technology Trends by Hospital Era

Era	Philosophy	Technology level	Data Management Tools	Data Management Methods
1960s	Process view of the world Data as by-product	Mainframes No networks	None	None
1970s	Process view of the world Data as by-product	First Minis First disk drives	First DBMSs	Structured analysis and design Data base administration
1980s	Holistic view of the world Data as common asset	PCs appear Department networks	PC DBMSs First distributed DBMSs First CASE tools	Data modeling Prototyping Relational theory Data administration
1990s	Holistic view of the world Data as strategic asset	Enterprise networks Internetworks PCs acquire most mainframe features	Heterogeneous distributed DBMSs ntegrated CASE tools	Object modeling Business process reengineering Sophisticated data policies

does not support the logic of the business. This happens when management cannot obtain answers to its questions, which, over time, are becoming more complex and integrative. Requests for data on "Total Patient Billings" have been replaced by requests for "Total Patient Billings minus Total Collections by Financial Class"; "Total Costs" have been replaced by "Total Costs by Physician by DRG"; "Total Procedures" have been replaced by "Total Procedures by Geographical Area." These cannot be answered because the data was not designed to be integrated. Top management understands how the business fits together, which is obvious from the questions. It is frustrated by the systems' inability to answer questions, but has no understanding of the reasons for this. Top management is thus unable to exercise effective leadership. Careers have been ruined over information systems. Until management has models and methods for dealing with the issues, they will be unable to effectively judge the performance of the IS department in the area of integration until after systems are implemented, at which point it becomes obvious that the systems cannot answer basic questions about the business.

Understanding

Top management needs to understand the nature and purpose of the data model. It codifies the business logic of the data. Models of management questions need to be developed, then linked to business processes at the level of the business cycle. Hospital administrators should not fear the use of a model. Models are used in every sphere of hospital activity: plant construction, physiology, finance, strategic planning, nursing, and so forth. Managers are expected to have familiarity with these models. Managers make decisions within the context of these models; they are not expected to understand every level of detail, but it is unthinkable that the executive would allow work to be done without a review of the models that underlie this work. When a question arises about space allocation within a new wing, managers discuss it using blueprints. When a financial decision needs to be made, the chart of accounts or the balance sheet is reviewed. When organizational decisions are being made, management refers to the organization chart.

The data model is just another model needed by managers who are required to perform in an increasingly complex world. The data model is literally a "blueprint" for the data. Just as the architectural drawings of a building show both the integrated totality and the different subsystems (electrical, telecommunications, fire and safety, furniture, etc.), so the data model shows the whole and the subsystems. Figure 5.7 shows the "big picture" of the data, which top management must demand from the IS department. The CEO approaches it from the "big picture" point of view. He/she deals with the stakeholders, and wants to know how the

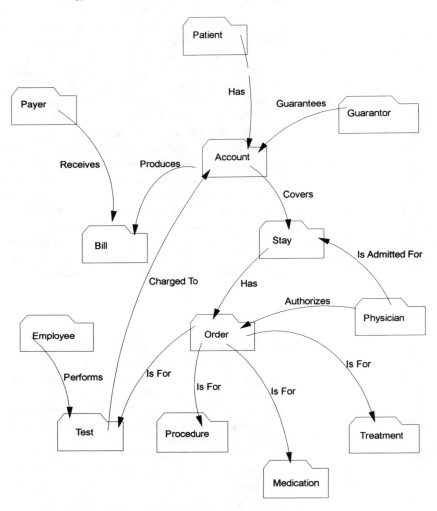

Figure 5.7 Executive blueprint for data.

data bases can help the hospital provide value to them. For example, do the data bases provide an integrated picture of the data to physicians? What can the information systems do for the Joint Commission on Accreditation of Healthcare Organizations (JCAHO)? What can they do to improve our relationships with large payers? What can they provide for the strategic plan and the Board of Trustees?

Much depends on the personality and style of the top executive. In many cases, the CEO may employ a trusted translator, such as a CIO or VP of information systems.

Leadership

Once executives have a way to pose questions and assimilate new material, they can make the difficult decisions required to align the data bases with the business. They will never be involved in detailed systems design, but they will have checklists of questions that can be put to the IS department to verify that the systems are moving in the direction of integration. For example, does the new system connect with the existing systems? Can one obtain an integrated report out of the systems? Can this integrated data be sent throughout the hospital to any and all interested parties? Armed with this strong appreciation of how the world of systems should be and can be, a CEO will be able to show leadership on related questions of systems planning, systems development, cost/benefit analysis, and other controls needed to ensure a fit between systems and the business. This will be discussed in greater detail in Chapters 6 and 7.

TECHNICAL DISCUSSION

The most important piece of the Data Architecture is the Data Model. It is the logical glue that holds together the Business Processes and the Technology that supports them. A logical view is necessary because both business processes and technology are dynamic. On the business side, new products are introduced, organizations are created and modified, and new policies and procedures are created and modified. On the technology side, computers are acquired and upgraded, new software is developed, new network segments are installed, and so forth. The link between the business processes and the technology is the *data*. The business processes use it, and the technology collects and distributes it. While all this change is occurring, the blueprint for the data—the Data Model—remains relatively stable. This concept is illustrated in Figure 5.8.

One cannot integrate systems physically until one can understand them logically. And one cannot understand them logically until one can model the data contained within them.

The "Data Architecture" consists of data blueprints and a set of policies and procedures that enforce their use. In particular, they are:

- The Data Model.
- Map between the Data Model and the physical information systems.
- Map between the business process and the Data Model.
- Policies and procedures for control.

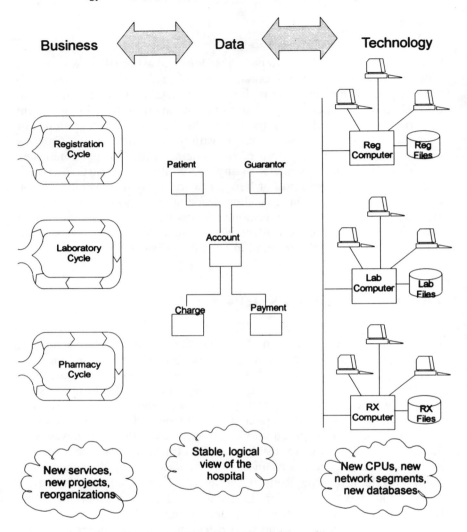

Figure 5.8 The integrating value of data.

When data is managed as a common resource, new control issues arise:

- Who owns what parts of the Physician data?
- Who controls the Charge Master? How should a department insert a new charge?
- Who owns what portions of the Patient data base?
- Who is responsible for maintaining and enforcing the data model?

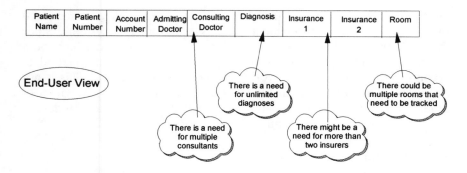

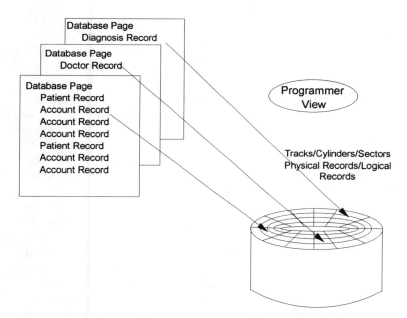

Figure 5.9 End-user view versus programmer view.

These issues should be handled by policies and procedures, budgeting and chargeback techniques, systems development techniques, and reward systems. (See Chapter 7: Control Architecture.)

Whether viewed from management's position or technology's position, hospitals act as though there is no underlying data model when they develop or acquire information systems. End users and managers jump to uninformed requirements (see Figure 5.9), and technical staff jump to physical file layouts. The challenge for the hospital is to take the business entities, which characterize the environment of hospital managers, and turn them into the data elements of physical computer systems. Since these are two antithetical ways of looking at the world, there must be a common ground—the data model. The end user wants to automate data according to his view of the world, as one long, flat record. This is not acceptable since the hospital's view is not served, nor are the views of other users. The remainder of this chapter is devoted to data modeling. This is the most important skill for integration.

Data Model

Definition of Data Model

A Data Model is the abstract graphic representation of a hospital's data. It represents those facts and objects that the hospital must track for management purposes. It includes things such as "Patient," "Order," "Test," "Charge." The Data Model accommodates both the global, or "enterprise" view of the data and at the same time the departmental, or "local" view. The local views are all subsets of the global view, and they are slanted by the department's function and place in the patient care process. For example, "lab tests" in the eyes of the Business Office represents those charges debited to a patient's account for the tests associated with a particular stay at the hospital. The Business Office person wants to relate this data to Financial Class and Insurer (Are these charges covered?), to the Charge Master (Is the charge coded correctly?), and to the Account (Is the charge posted to the correct account?). The Lab technician has a different view of the world. For him, "lab tests" represents the specimens and test results for a particular patient. The lab tech wants to relate this data to Medicines (Is the patient taking medication that could skew the readings?), Procedures (did he follow the correct lab procedure?), and Medical Record Number (Is this the correct patient?). There are many more "stakeholders" in lab tests, each with his own idiosyncratic view of the world. Nevertheless, they all work in the same hospital, as part of the same patient care process, and so the hospital, the "enterprise," is interested in all those views. Therefore, the global data model must accommodate all the "local" views. Each department has its own view of the data, a limited subset of the hospital's data. The Lab does not care about guarantor information; Registration does not care about market segments.

The data model is abstract because it portrays the *logical* entities and their relationships, not the mechanisms for their physical storage and retrieval. Most hospitals have more than one computer system, even if these systems are personal computers. The data will be distributed across multiple physical systems. Each computer supports a departmental view. The Lab computer will have Patient data, but only that data which interests Lab, and is structured according to Lab's world view. As a result, the data becomes partitioned, fragmented, and duplicated. And the mechanisms for this are different: flat files versus DBMS's; 4GL access versus Cobol and C; DOS versus MVS and VMS. And the nomenclature is different. The data model captures the business logic of the hospital's data. The challenge is to structure the physical systems, which house and distribute the data, so that they support the business logic.

How to Read a Data Model

There are several different techniques for drawing a data model. Two of the leading techniques are Bachmann diagrams and the ER models of Peter Chen. The technique employed in this book is based on a method called "IDEF1X." This acronym stands for "Integrated [Computer-Aided Manufacturing] Definition Method–1X." It was developed by D. Appleton Company for the U.S. Air Force, and is in the public domain. Figure 5.10 represents a fragment of a data model for the Registration function. It shows the business structure for data that is important to the hospital: Patient, Insurer, Stay, Account, and Physician.

Entity: Represented by rectangles. An Entity is something about which the hospital keeps data. An Entity can be a person, place, activity, thing, or event. Typical hospital entities are patient, facility, procedure, supply item, charge, diagnosis, employee, and so on.

Relationship: Represented by lines and dots. A Relationship is a meaningful connection between two entities. For example, we want to know what Diagnoses are made by a Physician; how many Visits a Patient has had; how many Accounts are the responsibility of a Guarantor; and so on. The dots on the lines indicate "cardinality," that is, how many occurrences of one entity can be associated with the other entity. For example, the line connecting Patient with Account states: A given Account will be for one and only one Patient; a given Patient can have many Accounts. These relationships express business rules. The labels on the lines indicate the name of the relationship. They only show one side of the relationship and they are read in the direction from the independent entity (the entity without the dot).

Key Attribute: The text inside the Entity symbol represents the "attributes" or characteristics of that Entity. For example, a Patient has such attributes as Name, Weight, Date of Birth, and so on. Some attributes serve to uniquely identify each occurrence of a particular entity. They are called "key attributes" and are indicated by a horizontal line drawn underneath. For example, the key attribute of Patient is Medical Record Number (MRN), because it uniquely identifies each instance of patient.

---

[1] For further discussion of IDEF1X, see Mary Loomis, *The Database Book*, New York: MacMillan, 1987, and Thomas A. Bruce, *Designing Quality Databases with IDEF1X Information Models*, New York: Dorset House Publishing, 1992.

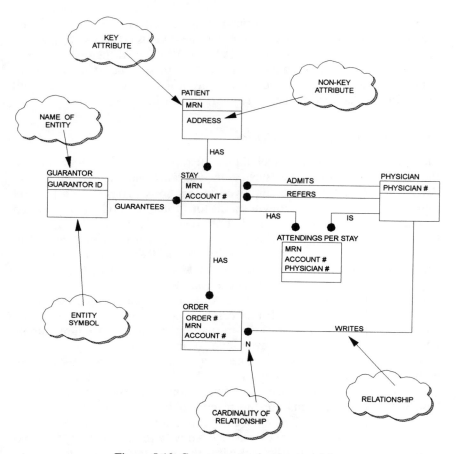

Figure 5.10 Components of a data model.

Non-key attributes are any characteristics of the entity which do not serve to identify it. Figure 5.10 can be read in the following way:

> A patient can have many stays. Each stay must have a guarantor. Each stay must have an admitting physician. There may be a referring physician. The stay may have many orders. An order cannot be created, unless it can be related to a stay.

How to Construct a Data Model

The are three different levels, or phases, of a data model:

1. *Entity-Relationship model.* This is used for high-level planning. As its name suggests, this model consists just of entities and relationships.

2. *Key-based model*. In this model, the relationships are much more precise, and the entities are indentified by their key attributes. This model can be used for design.

3. *Fully attributed model*. This model contains all of the non-key attributes of the entities. This model can be used for implementation.

The approach is top-down: First, construct a high-level model, then gradually develop a more detailed one. Eventually, the model can be mapped into a data distribution system that will consist of a network and individual file systems and/or data bases. The following sections will concentrate on developing the data model behind a local view for a single department—Diagnostic Imaging. (At the end of this chapter there will be some comments on integrating department views into an enterprise view.)

1. Entity-Relationship Model

The Entity-Relationship (E-R) model is the first level of detail. It is also called the Data Planning Model. For an entire hospital, the Data Planning Model consists of approximately fifty entities. For a given department, it might consist of ten to twelve entities. It presents a high-level view of the major data categories. It is constructed during systems planning or in the first phase of requirements definition for a particular application.

1.1 Record the Business Views

As a way of getting started, assemble a group of the department's managers, together with the department head. Ask each person to develop a list of six major objectives, six major measures of success, and six major activities. This is good for developing the scope. For example:

The major objective of the radiology department is to provide high-quality diagnostic imaging for the hospital's patients. Another goal is to provide cost-effective treatment. A third goal is patient satisfaction. A fourth goal is to attract and retain skilled professionals.

The major measures of success are: numbers of X-rays performed weekly, amount of employee turnover, conformance to the department's budget for both costs and revenues, conformance to pre-established schedules, results of patient satisfaction surveys.

The major activities are: scheduling of physicians and patients, maintenance of the equipment, taking of X-rays, development and storage of X-rays, recording and reconciling charges to patient accounts.

Another way to assemble this scoping information is to obtain departmental documents such as a mission statement, an organization chart, procedures manual, or monthly management reports.

1.2 Develop Candidate Entities

After recording the managers' statements, examine them for data entities. Do this by underlining the nouns. An entity is defined as any person, place, object, or event about which the hospital must keep data. At this point the underlined nouns are "candidate entities": they will later undergo validation and refinement. Some will be discarded; others will be expanded; still others will be redefined. The candidate entities are italicized in the following paragraphs.

> The major objective of the radiology *department* is to provide high-quality diagnostic *imaging* for the hospital's *patients*. Another goal is to provide cost-effective *treatment*. A third goal is patient *satisfaction*. A fourth goal is to attract and retain skilled *professionals*.
>
> The major *measures* of success are: numbers of *X-rays* performed weekly, amount of employee *turnover*, conformance to the department's *budget* for both *costs* and *revenues*, conformance to preestablished *schedules*, results of patient satisfaction *surveys*.
>
> The major activities are: scheduling of *physicians* and *patients*, *maintenance* of the *equipment*, taking of *X-rays*, *development* and *storage* of X-rays; recording and reconciling *charges* to patient *accounts*.

1.3 Test for Valid Entities

In order to be judged an entity in the data model, the candidate entity must pass the following tests:

1. It must be a person, place, thing, or event. Adjectives, such as "green" or "efficient," do not pass this test. However, abstract nouns that represent activities ("maintenance") or events ("charge") do qualify as entities.

2. It must represent a class or a set of objects. For example, Emergency Room is not a set containing multiple members; it is one single location.

3. Each instance of the class must be uniquely identifiable. It must have a set of attributes that serve to identify it.

Table 5.3 contains the entities that pass the tests.

1.4 Determine the Relationships among Entities

Next, determine the relationships that hold among the entities that have been identified. This can be done by brainstorming, or, in a more struc-

Table 5.3 Evaluation of Candidate Entities

Candidate entity	Valid entity	Comment
Department	Yes	An entity; it is a thing; it represents a class of object; each one is uniquely identifiable (through department name or department number).
Hospital	No	Not an entity, because there is only one instance for this item; that is, there is only one hospital in question (the situation would be different with a chain of hospitals).
Patient	Yes	An entity; it represents a class of persons; each Patient is uniquely identifiable (through Medical Record Number).
Quality	No	Not an entity; it is an abstract noun (typically, abstract nouns do not qualify as entities unless they represent activities); it does not represent a class of objects (one instance of "quality" cannot be differentiated from another).
Professional	Yes	An entity; it represents a class of persons; each instance can be uniquely identified (through SSN or Employee ID).
Measure	Yes	An entity (in its nominal meaning); it represents a class of things; each measure can be uniquely identified.
X-ray	Yes	An entity; it represents a class of things; each X-ray can be uniquely identified (through Sequence Number).
Budget	Yes	An entity; it represents a class of things; each budget can be uniquely identified (through department number and Budget Version Number, for example).
Cost	Yes	An entity (perhaps); it represents a class of things; each cost can be uniquely identified (through Cost Number or Account Number).
Revenue	No	Not an entity; it does not represent a class of things; one revenue cannot be distinguished from another revenue.
Schedule	No	Not an entity; at first glance it appears to represent a class of things; later analysis will reveal that it is nothing more than a report.
Account	Yes	An entity.
Physician	Yes	An entity (perhaps a subcategory of Professional).
Equipment	Yes	An entity; it represents a class of things; each instance can be uniquely identified through Fixed Asset Number.
Charge	Yes	An entity; it represents a class of events; each instance can be uniquely identified through Product Code, Account Number, and Date.

tured fashion, by constructing a matrix and comparing each entity to all the others (see Figure 5.11). Fill in the cells in either half of the matrix by naming the relationships among the intersecting entities. When associating entities, the analyst will find other entities. The analyst needs to ask, for example: "What is the relationship between Patient and Account?" The user might answer: "Before the registration clerk may admit the patient and open a new account, the clerk must have a valid insurer. If the

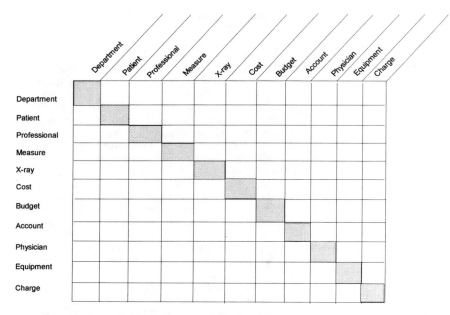

Figure 5.11 Entity matrix for establishing relationships.

patient does not have insurance, the clerk must contact his supervisor for authorization of the admission." Some of the relationships may be found in official statements of hospital policy.

The data modeler must exercise judgment and restraint when setting up relationships, and choose only the most immediate, direct relationships. In a rationally organized system (of which Radiology is an example), everything is related to everything else, however remotely. Many novice data modelers connect everything to everything else, using trivial relationships. For example, one might try to set up a direct relationship between Patient and Equipment: "A patient is treated with a piece of equipment." Subsequent analysis will show that this is an indirect relationship.

1.5 Develop the Business Statements and Cardinality

The relationships must be turned into "business statements," which are English-language statements explaining the nature of the relationship and expressing the cardinality. Indeed, the business statements actually represent statements of business policy. Each business statement has two parts, one for each end of the relationship:

Department-Patient

- A given Department has 0/1/many Patients.
- A given Patient stays in 0/1/many Departments.

Department-Professional

- A given Department has 0/1/many Professionals.
- A given Professional works in 0/1/many Departments.

Restating relationships as business statements allows end users to more effectively validate the truth of the statement. Let's assume that we have established a relationship between Patient and Account.

- A given patient can have 0/1/many accounts;
- A given account is for one and only one patient.

The resulting business statement appears correct to the analyst, but the end user, upon reading the relationship in both directions, might be prompted to recall a situation that contradicts the business statement: The hospital has something called an "institutional account," which collects the charges of multiple patients who are the patients of *other* hospitals sent for a specialized outpatient service. This will cause the model to be corrected through the addition of another entity, Institutional Account. We are interested in both naming and understanding the structure of the relationships. Wherever a relationship has "0/1/many" as its cardinality, we place a dot ("●") on that end. If the cardinality is a specific number, the dot should be labeled with that number. For example, a year contains *twelve* months.

When a hospital purchases an HIS from a vendor, it is frequently cardinality that causes misalignment between the system's model and the hospital's business model. How many attending physicians may a patient have? Usually one is enough, but not in a tertiary-care hospital. How many consulting physicians are enough? Usually two or three, but not in a teaching hospital. If a hospital's policy is that attendings (students) rotate to another service after a month, and if a patient stays longer than a month, then the system does not conform with hospital policy. The hospital must then decide whether it should change its policies. But in many cases, these policies are part of the business strategy or result from the nature of the organization, and cannot be changed. Then the hospital has to jury-rig its record-keeping procedures to accommodate the system, keeping a manual record of the first attending. This can also lead to statistical inaccuracies.

1.6 Build the Graphic E-R Model

In parallel with the business statements, draw a model using the graphic conventions defined on the preceding pages. Figure 5.12 can be read in the following way:

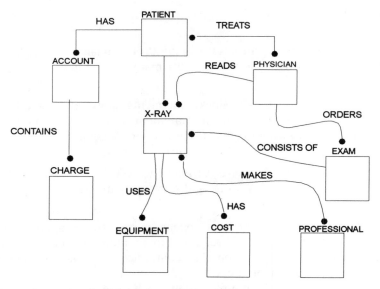

Figure 5.12 Entity-relationship model.

A patient can have many accounts. A given account is for one and only one patient. A patient is treated by 0/1/many physicians. A physician treats 0/1/many patients, and so forth.

It can be seen that some entities are independent, while other entities cannot exist alone. For example, an account cannot be created unless there is a patient. This is called "existence dependence." But a patient can exist whether or not there is an account.

All relationships must be labeled. Note that a relationship can be read either forward or backward, but that the wording may change, based on the direction: a Patient *has* an Account; an Account *is for* a Patient. Remember to label the lines for Cardinality. If one end of the relationship is unity, then it is not labeled with a dot. A single dot indicates 0/1/many occurrences of the dependent entity.

Note that some relationships are "many-to-many" (Patient:Physician and X-ray:Professional). Such relationships need to be reworked to remove the "many" from one of the ends. This is done at the next level of model—the Key-based Model.

1.7 Add Textual Definitions and Comments

A complete Data Model also requires definitions and any relevant commentary. Each entity and the relationships in which it participates must be defined in a dictionary, whether manual or automated. The planning model contains a manageable number of entities, but subsequent models will swell the number of entities to 50–100 per department. The diagram, by itself, has great communication and analytical value, but it cannot convey all that is known about the data.

It should be emphasized that this process, like any analytical process, is an iterative one. By looking at this model, one can see the scoping value of it.

2. Key-based Model

The Entity-Relationship Model is used for high-level planning, but not for implementation. The Key-based Model contains the details that show how the pieces fit together. In this phase, the modeler begins to perform many of the activities associated with "normalization." He determines the "primary key" for each entity, resolves many-to-many relationships, and so on. The key-based model for a department should be two to five times larger than the data planning model. Obviously, this depends on the scope of the data planning model. The number of entities grows as each step is performed.

2.1 Resolve Many-to-many Relationships

Two sets of entities in the Data Planning Model shown in Figure 5.12 participate in a many-to-many relationship. Most many-to-many relationships can be resolved by inserting a third entity between the two entities in question. Figure 5.13 shows Patient:Physician being resolved by inserting a treatment entity (Patient Treated by Physician). The result reads as, "A patient gets 0/1/many treatments, each provided by a single physician; a physician provides 0/1/many treatments, each given to a single patient." The resolution of X-ray:Professional is similar. It requires the creation of an entity called "X-ray Participant."

2.2 Determine the Primary Key for Each Entity

Figure 5.14 shows the primary key inserted for each entity. The primary key uniquely identifies each instance of an entity, and is indicated by drawing a line under it. It may consist of more than one attribute. For example, the primary key of Patient might be Medical Record Number, while the primary key of Visit might be Medical Record Number plus Admit Date. There may be alternate keys—other attributes that also uniquely identify each instance of the entity (for example, SSN for Patient).

In this process, the data modeler will frequently find that traditional ID numbers and keys, which appear to be single identifiers, are really the concatenation of several things. For example, Visit Number might equal MRN + Date. It should be emphasized that the term "primary key" refers to the logical identification of the entity. It has nothing to do with

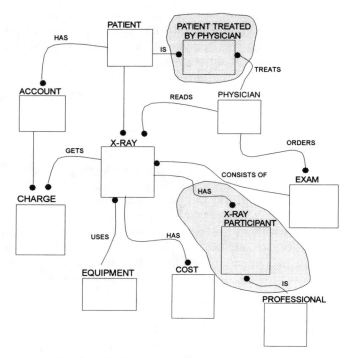

Figure 5.13 Resolution of N:N relationships.

the indexing methods employed within a given system for physically accessing and retrieving records. (It should also be emphasized that Figure 5.14 is just a working model. It has inaccuracies, which will be removed throughout the process of modeling, and simplifications for the sake of exposition.)

Table 5.4 summarizes the entities and their key attributes discovered so far. In general, the independent entities have fewer attributes in their primary key. This is natural, since they may exist independently of any other entity. There are other entities that depend on events or transactions. For example, a charging event is needed for Charge to come into existence, linking a Service with an Account; a registration event is needed to create an Account, which must be linked to a Patient.

2.3 Migrate Primary Key into Dependent Entities

After primary keys are assigned, they must be migrated "downward" from the independent entity to the dependent entity. Figure 5.15 highlights the migrated keys. A key can migrate across many entities. If it winds up in a key position, it must be migrated to the next dependent entity. It continues to migrate into dependent entities, until it winds up in

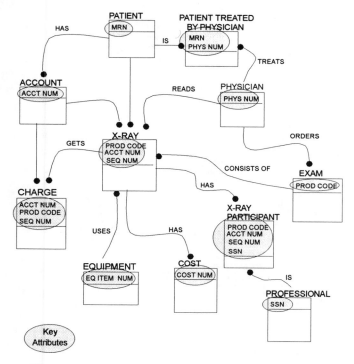

Figure 5.14 Primary key attributes inserted into model.

Table 5.4 Entities and Their Key Attributes

Entity	Added	Key attribute(s)
Patient		Medical Record Number
Patient Treated by Physician	Yes	Medical Record Number
		Physician Number
Physician		Physician Number
Account		Account Number
Charge		Account Number
		Product Code
		Sequence Number
X-ray		Product Code
		Account Number
		Sequence Number
X-ray Participant	Yes	Product Code
		Account Number
		Sequence Number
		Social Security Number
Exam		Product Code
Equipment		Equipment Item Number
Cost		Cost Number
Professional		Social Security Number

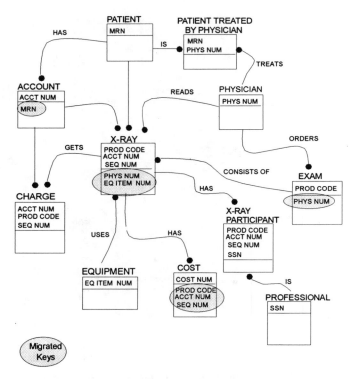

Figure 5.15 Migration of key attributes.

a non-key position. This can be seen in the entities Account, X-ray, and X-ray Participant. Account Number migrates down into X-ray, where it winds up in a key position. It migrates downward again, into X-ray Participant. There are no more dependent entities, so migration stops with X-ray Participant. With Patient and Account, the primary key moves into a non-key position, so its migration stops when it gets to Account.

Sometimes the very process of defining the primary key for a dependent entity will result in placing the migrating key in key position. If this happens, the key should not be duplicated in the migration step. For example, Acct Num would not be migrated from Account into Charge because it already occurs as a result of defining the Key of Charge.

Recall that the primary key is denoted by a line drawn under it across the entity symbol. The secondary key is placed below this line. Recall that an independent entity is an entity that is on the singular end of a relationship; a dependent entity is on the "●" end of the relationship. This has significance for data integrity: A dependent entity cannot be created if there is no existing independent entity on the other end of the relationship. For example, a hospital (and by extension, its computer system) should prevent the creation of a patient account if there is no patient for it. Conversely, a Patient entity can be created without the need to have a Patient Account.

2.4 Test for Repeating Groups

For each of the migrated keys, the analyst must ask whether it can have multiple values. It turns out that some accounts can have multiple values for MRN, because they can have multiple patients associated with them. These are the "institutional" accounts discussed earlier. (If a feature needing to be normalized is not discovered in one step of the methodology, it will be discovered in another.) This hospital provides Diagnostic Imaging services to the patients of other hospitals in the area. This requires the establishment of an Institutional Account entity, which has a many-to-many relationship with Patient, which is then resolved with the "Patient on Institutional Account" entity and which then undergoes all the tests discussed so far, highlighted in Figure 5.16.

2.5 Test for Null Values

For each of the migrated keys, one must ask whether it can ever have no value. When the "X-ray" entity is created, there may be no value for Physician Number. This is because there is a delay between the taking of the X-ray and the reading of it by the physician. This requires an additional entity, called "Read X-ray." A Read X-ray will always have a value for Physician Number. See Figure 5.16.

2.6 Reformulate the Business Rules

The model has changed significantly, so the business rules must be restated. The business rules have a technical reading and a business reading. The business reading represents the business implications.

Patient: Account
Technical: A given Patient has 0/1/many Accounts; a given Account has
              one and only one Patient.
Business: You may set up a Patient in the data base without having an
              Account for it; in order to set up an Account in the data
              base, you must assign it to a Patient.

Sometimes, there is a simple two-entity relationship, as in Patient and Account. In other cases, a given entity can participate in relationships with a rather large number of other entities.

X-ray: Patient, Physician, Charge, Equipment, Cost, Professional, Exam
Technical: 1   A given Patient has 0/1/many X-rays; a given X-ray has
                  one and only one Patient.

Business: 1   You may set up a Patient in the data base without having any X-rays for it; when you record an X-ray, you must have a Patient for it.

Technical: 2   A given Physician reads 0/1/many X-rays; a given X-ray is read by one and only one Physician.

Business: 2   When you set up a Physician in the data base, you do not need to have an X-ray for her/him; when you record an X-ray, there must be a Physician who reads it.

Technical: 3   A given X-ray has 0/1 Charges; a given Charge is for one and only one X-ray.

Business: 3   When you record an X-ray, there may or may not be a Charge; when you record a Charge, it must be assigned to an X-ray.

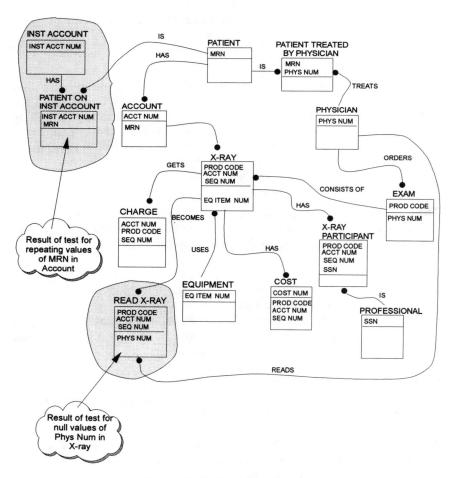

Figure 5.16 Revised model.

Many of these relationships are existence dependent. The entity on the singularity end of the relationship may exist without a corresponding entity on the 0/1/many end; conversely, the entity on the 0/1/many end may not exist without having an entity on the other end. You may have a Patient without an Account, and an Account without a Charge. Any relationship can be read in two directions. Sometimes, the phrasing will be different: "A Patient has 0/1/many Accounts," but "an Account is for one and only one Patient." In most cases, the models in this book contain relationship labels expressing the independent end of the relationship.

2.7 Other Issues

The analyst needs to repeatedly check the relationships and business rules. It sometimes turns out that changes to the model cause some of the existing relationships to become redundant. For example, Patient:X-ray is now redundant, since X-ray can be linked to Patient through Account. The relationship Account:Charge also turns out to be redundant, since a Charge can be associated with its Account through X-ray.

As the analyst tests the business rules, he will find examples that contradict the initial statements. For example, some hospitals provide outpatient services to patients of other hospitals. Rather than set up a separate account for each external patient, they use a group account to handle all the charges. If you expect the information system to accommodate this, then you need to change the model. In addition, you may realize that your hospital requires that you track multiple employees for a given X-ray, or multiple Physicians reading a given X-ray. While there are generic patterns of data relationships, there is no "monolithic" hospital data model.

As work on the model proceeds, other insights occur. Someone may note that the Physician can order more services than just X-rays, and that X-ray is really a category of Service; or that not all patients get admitted, and so there are different categories of Patient (Inpatient, Outpatient, Day Surgery, etc.). Discovery of these categories results naturally from the modeling techniques. Figure 5.17 shows a new entity, Service, which is subcategorized into Medicine, X-ray Exam, and Lab Test. The X-ray exam may consist of more than one shot (X-ray). These individual X-rays get Charges.

Eventually, it would be shown that each of these subcategories has its own set of distinct relationships; they might also have different non-key attributes. For example, Lab Test would have a relationship with Specimen, or Medicine would have non-key attributes concerning allergies. However, they all have the same primary key as the generic entity, Service, because they are all types of Service. They are distinguished by a "discriminator" attribute (Service Type). The relationship reads the following way: A Service may be either a Medicine, an X-ray Exam, or a Lab Test; a Medicine is a type of Service; an X-ray Exam is a type of

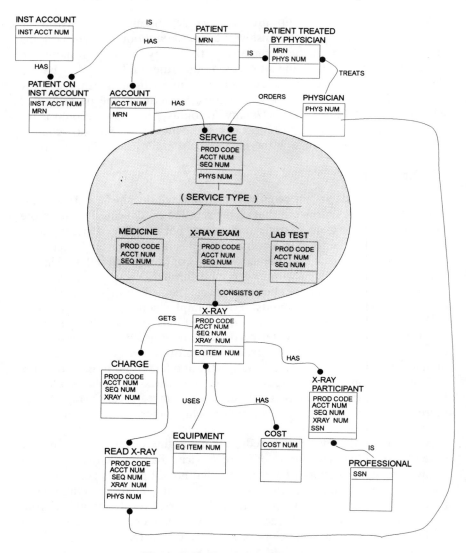

Figure 5.17 Category relationship.

Service; a Lab Test is a type of Service. Frequently, one finds these category relationships when one tries to reconcile different departmental views into an enterprise model. These general relationships subsume the more specific, departmental view. This will subsequently be discovered when the analyst tries to insert all the non-key attributes and applies the tests.

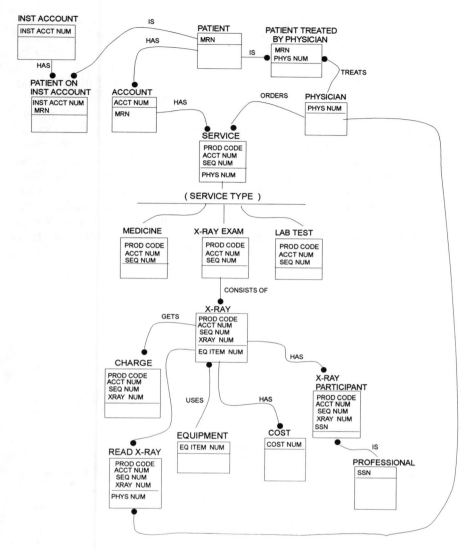

Figure 5.18 Final version of key-based model.

2.8 Redraw Model

Figure 5.18 presents the final version of the Key-based Model. At this point, the overall logical structure of the Diagnostic Imaging data is apparent, and the hospital can begin to define how the DI system fits with existing information systems. A good place to start is with the independent entities. It is clear that Patient, Professional, Physician, Cost, and

Equipment will be in multiple systems. As a matter of fact, other systems will keep much more data about these entities than will the DI system. For example the registration system will have *all* the patient demographics and insurance data.

Nevertheless, if the key attributes are comparable, and if access and distribution mechanisms are in place, then all patient data are accessible through the key attributes Medical Record Number and Account Number. The key attributes are all that is necessary to obtain an integrated view of the data. The same holds for Fixed Assets. It contains depreciation schedules and preventive maintenance schedules for the equipment that is used by the DI staff and it is accessed by Equipment Item Number. The Clinical Information System may hold real-time data on patient vital signs, and it will be accessible through Medical Record Number. The Medical Staff Management system holds statistics on number of X-rays performed by medical staff members, for credentialing purposes. It is accessible through Physician Number. See Figure 5.19.

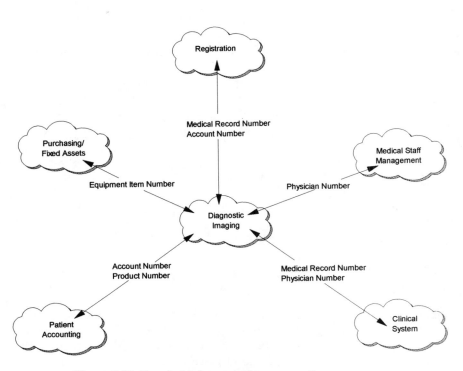

Figure 5.19 Keys hold data together across diverse systems.

3. Fully Attributed Model

A "fully attributed" data model has the following characteristics:

- All non-key attributes are defined for each entity (e.g., attributes such as Date of Birth or Sex, for Patient).
- All attributes that have multiple values have been broken down into separate entities. For example, a Diagnosis attribute will probably be reanalyzed into a Diagnosis entity.
- Within an entity, all non-key attributes must depend exclusively on the primary key.
- There must be no dependencies among non-key attributes.
- No attributes may have a null value.

The above are the characteristics of a "Third Normal Form," which is generally considered to be the minimum amount of logical structure needed to design a physical data base. The method used to arrive at this Third Normal Form has been "top-down." Many of the traditional systems analysis methodologies use a "bottom up" approach, which requires extensive analysis of the details of documents and record layouts. In these methodologies it is harder to involve the end user, since the analysis starts off at too detailed a level.

The Data Planning Model for a department has around ten entities. The key-based model is two to five times larger; the fully attributed model is another two to five times larger than the key-based model. Thus, for a single department, if the modeler starts with ten entities in the Data Planning Model, he or she will eventually have a fully attributed model of 40 to 250 entities, but probably closer to 200 on the average. If a hospital has 30 departments, the number of entities in the enterprise data model could easily reach 5,000.

3.1 Insert Non-Key Attributes

All the non-key attributes for each entity must be defined. For the sake of exposition, however, this chapter does not provide an exhaustive listing of non-key attributes for each entity. Instead, it uses a representative number of non-key attributes, contained in Table 5.5. The new data model is presented in Figure 5.20, with non-key attributes highlighted. This model shows no structural changes or expansion yet. This will occur when the non-key attributes undergo a series of tests similar to those performed in Section 2.

3.2 Separate Repeating Values

Any attribute that can have multiple values must be broken down into a separate entity. Several attributes can have repeating values. They are

Table 5.5 "Representative" Non-key Attributes

Entity	Non-key Attributes
Patient	Date of Birth
	Age
	Admit Date
	Admitting Physician
	Room Number
Account	Balance
Physician	Physician Name
	Specialty
Service	Date Ordered
	Date Rendered
X-ray Exam	Price
Charge	Date Charged
X-ray Participant	Employee Name
Read X-ray	Checkout Date
	Return Date
	Comments

Admit Date (in Patient), Room Number (in Patient), and Price (in X-ray Exam). A given patient may be admitted multiple times; for a given stay, a patient may have multiple rooms; over time, a given exam may have more than one price. This results in the creation of three additional entities: Room, X-ray Exam Price, and Admitted Patient. One might want to put Admit Date into Account, but this would fail the null value test, since one can set up an Account without having a value for Admit Date. It also turns out that Room has a many-to-many relationship with Admitted Patient (see Figure 5.21). One could have connected Room with Patient, but this would not be sufficient, since the hospital needs to track the Room by each of the Patient's stays.

In reality, few information systems allow the hospital to record multiple rooms for a given stay, so they are kept in manual records. This, of course, depends on how the hospital wants to run itself. Another issue arises: Is the hospital willing to set up the procedures and controls for this data? If the hospital says it needs to have multiple rooms per stay, then it must also make a commitment to record that data.

The concept of "Schedule" is interesting. Many readers are liable to ask about the existence of a Schedule entity. Schedule is actually a report, not an entity. It has many attributes that have repeating values. Further analysis causes it to be replaced by an entity called Scheduled Event, which is the nexus of Room, Date, Time, Equipment Item, Service, and Staff. A "Schedule" is thus merely a report that contains the multiple Scheduled Events. Novice data modelers frequently make the mistake of modeling a physical report rather than its underlying data.

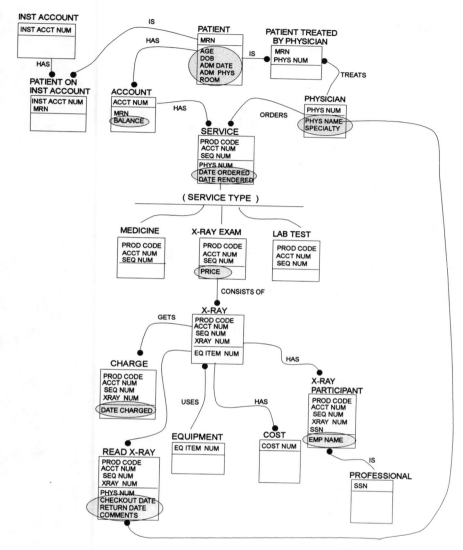

Figure 5.20 Model with non-key attributes.

3.3 Test for Null Values

Any attribute that can have a null value should be moved out into a separate entity. Figure 5.22a highlights the attributes that have null values. Figure 5.22b shows the resulting changes to the model. Date Rendered in the entity Service will have a null value until the service

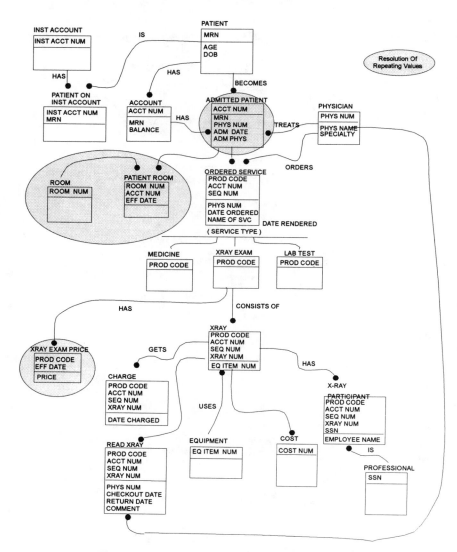

Figure 5.21 Model expanded for repeating values.

is provided, so it is moved into a separate entity, called "Rendered Service," and "Service" is renamed "Ordered Service" to make its meaning clearer. The entity "Read X-ray" initially will have no value for Return Date, so another entity is created to accommodate the checkout activity. Not every checked-out X-ray will have an interpreting physician; this indicates the need for yet another entity. Many such cases turn out to represent the stages through which an entity proceeds. A good example is

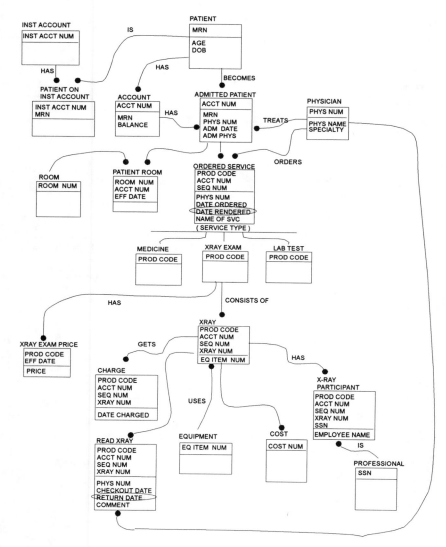

Figure 5.22a Null value problems.

the entity Order. First, there is an Order, then a Validated Order, then a
Filled Order, and finally a Charged Order. An Order can take a different
path and wind up becoming a Canceled Order (not reflected in the
model). Each time a new entity is identified, the data modeler must
repeat the steps of key migration, testing for repeating values, and testing
for nulls.

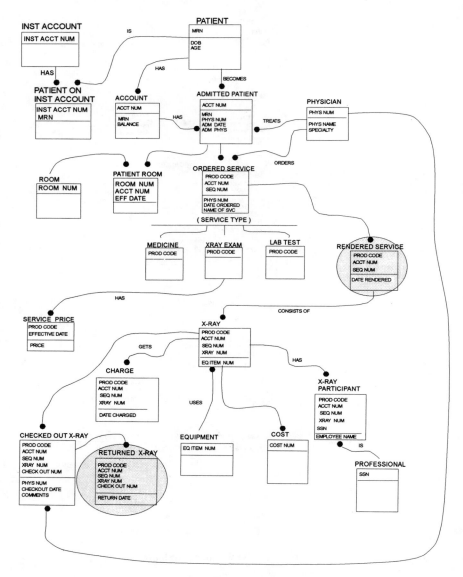

Figure 5.22b Resolution of null values.

3.4 Test for Dependencies

Two major tests remain. Within an entity, each non-key attribute must depend completely on the *full* key. If it depends on only a portion of the key it does not belong in the entity, and a new "home" must be found for it. For example, Name of Service depends solely on Product Code. The other portions of the key, Account Number and Sequence Number are irrelevant. This means that we must find another entity to house Name of Service. This entity is called "Service." Notice that we have just established the existence of the master file that provides the general information about the service, which would not be retained in each individual detail record. The same holds for "Employee Name" in X-ray Participant. It depends solely on SSN, and so it must be moved into the entity called "Professional" (Figure 5.23a).

The second test is for dependencies among/between non-key attributes. If one non-key attribute can be calculated from another, then it should not be included in the logical data model. For example, "Age" in the Patient entity can be calculated from Birth Date. And "Balance" in the entity Account can be calculated from the Price of each rendered service and any discounts that have been agreed upon. This should not be included in the logical data model. For performance reasons, Age may be stored as a field, rather than recalculated each time the patient record is retrieved during the stay. This will be part of the map from the data model to the physical data structures. See Figure 5.23b.

3.5 Review the Relationships

The new entities and relationships that arise as a result of these tests must be reviewed for correctness. Further examination of Physician and Admitted Patient prompts the insight that there are multiple relationships between the two entities: a Physician can "admit" a Patient; he can "attend" the Patient; and he can "consult" on the Patient. In addition, it turns out that the relationship between Patient and Admitted Patient is redundant, since Admitted Patient can be connected to Patient through Account. This is shown in Figure 5.24. Eventually, it would be discovered that there can be multiple values for Patient Name, causing it to be broken down as a separate entity, and showing the underpinnings of a physical Master Patient Index.

3.6 Update the Definitions and Commentary

Make sure that you have all the entities, and be sure to update all definitions and other comments to the model. A complete data model should be well documented. There are now many CASE tools to assist with drawing the models, maintaining the definitions, and converting the logical design into a physical data base design. The lack of tools used to be a serious impediment to data modeling. The models quickly become unmanageable without electronic support. They are too large and complex to either comprehend or change.

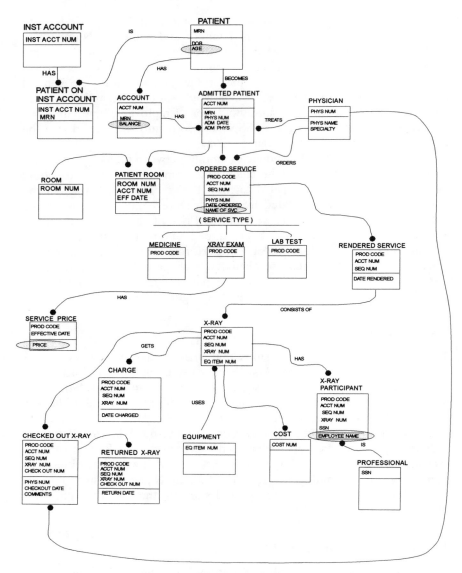

Figure 5.23a Problems with attribute dependencies.

3.7 Redraw the Model

After all the tests have been performed, the model is redrawn (Figure 5.25). It bears repeating that Figure 5.25 represents a particular way of managing a hospital. It requires only a single Attending Physician per Patient. Frequently, in a tertiary-care teaching setting there are multiple

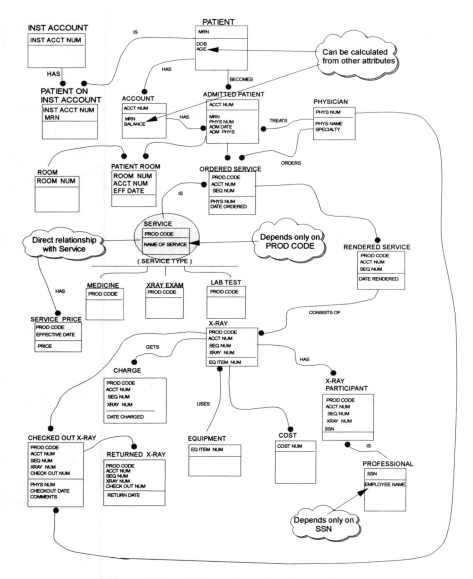

Figure 5.23b Attribute dependencies resolved.

Attending Physicians, due to lengthy stays and rotation of residents. On the other hand, the model does support multiple Consulting Physicians per Patient. Not all hospitals need that. This model also supports Institutional Accounts, which probably are not required by most hospitals. In addition, it specifies that the service is charged only after it is performed.

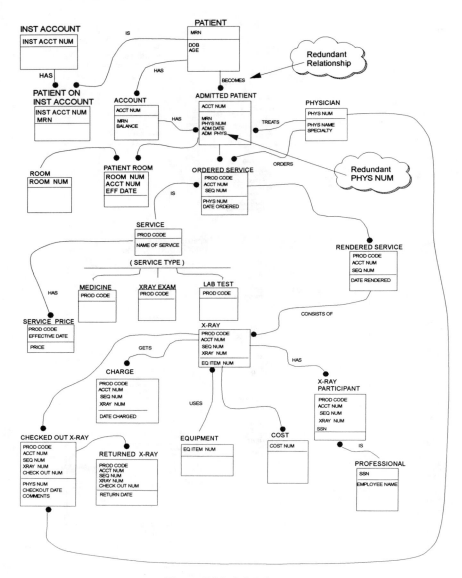

Figure 5.24 Other issues.

If a hospital has a manual business process that records a charge when the order is created, there will be a conflict. Finally, this model supports the participation of multiple people in a single exam.

Whether explicit or not, every HIS vendor has a data model underlying his/her system. This model may or may not match the business model of a

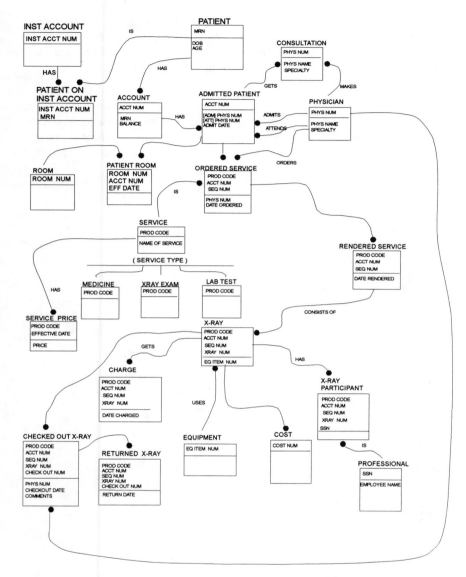

Figure 5.25 Final version of fully-attributed model.

given hospital. This lack of fit may have severe operational impacts. As a general rule, the more N:N relationships supported by the vendor, the better (e.g., Consultation and Attending Physician). An N:N relationship can always support a 1:N business model, but a 1:N relationship cannot support a N:N business model. The problem is that, for performance reasons, vendors try to pack as much data as they can into a single record or record segment, and this prevents effective support of N:N relationships. On the other hand, if one supports N:N relationships, this will require additional tables, and this will impact performance.

3.8 Validate the Model

There needs to be a final validation of the model by end users, to ensure accuracy and completeness. This can be done in two different ways: (1) The modeler and end user review the data model and the commentary

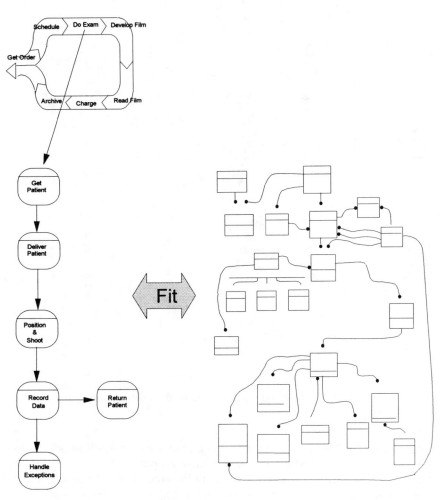

Figure 5.26 Validation of data model vis-à-vis activity model.

together; this is very abstract; and (2) the user and the analyst map the data model back to the flow diagrams of the business architecture. This latter technique compensates for the abstractness of the data model. Recall the three-part model presented in Figure 5.8, which shows the data architecture mediating between the Business Architecture and the Technical Architecture.

This technique is illustrated in Figure 5.26 using the business activity of Do Exam. Each of the tasks on the flow diagram activities within the cycle is reviewed for its data requirements, and these requirements are matched to the entities and attributes of the data model. This checks for the completeness of the model in terms of entities and attributes.

After this, the modeler validates the goodness of the relationships by taking the inquiry and reporting requirements and navigating the paths through the data model to determine whether it accommodates the inquiry and reporting requirements. In general, the paths for queries for decision support will be much more complex than those for operational transactions.

- What medicines was the patient taking when this X-ray was shot?
- Which physician ordered the most X-rays in a given month?
- What costs are incurred by physician X when treating a particular diagnosis as opposed to physician Y?
- Have all X-rays taken during the past two weeks been interpreted?
- A recall has been issued for a particular type of equipment. Which patients have been treated with it during the past month?

Table 5.6 explains how one would navigate the model to accommodate the above reporting requirements.

4. Map to a Specific DBMS or File Management System

The fully attributed model is a *logical* model, and it must be converted into a physical Data Base Management System, with specific record structures, storage mechanisms, and access strategies, including indexes. Any number of technologies could be used: relational DBMS's, hierarchical DBMS's, a MUMPS file system, other file management systems like IBM's VSAM and DEC's RMS. The ease with which these DBMS's can be made to behave so that they fit the business model will vary. The model could be converted straightforwardly into a relational DBMS, with each entity being mapped directly into a table (although most RDMS's do not enforce the integrity constraints of the model). With network data base management systems the mapping is more complex, and this clearly shows the need for a logical design. The logical model could be mapped to stand-alone files, but then all of the relationships would have to be managed by the application programs instead of the DBMS software. The

Table 5.6 Data Model Navigation to Answer Queries

Query	Path through the data base
What medicines was the patient taking when this X-ray was shot?	1. X-RAY → RENDERED SERVICE 2a. RENDERED SERVICE → SERVICE 2b. RENDERED SERVICE → ACCOUNT 3a. SERVICE → MEDICINE 3b. ACCOUNT → PATIENT 4. List patient data and the medicines
Which physician ordered the most X-rays in a given month?	1. X-RAY EXAM → ORDERED SERVICE 2. ORDERED SERVICE → PHYSICIAN 3. List the physicians
What costs are incurred by physician X when treating a particular diagnosis as opposed to physician Y?	1. PHYSICIAN → ORDERED SERVICE 2. ORDERED SERVICE → SERVICE 3a. SERVICE → MEDICINE 3b. SERVICE → X-RAY EXAM 3c. SERVICE → LAB TEST 4. Count costs for each physician
Have all X-rays taken during the past 2 weeks been interpreted?	1. SERVICE → RENDERED SERVICE 2. RENDERED SERVICE → X-RAY 3. X-RAY → CHECKED OUT X-RAY 4. CHECKED OUT X-RAY → RETURNED X-RAY 5. List and count all X-rays that have not been interpreted
A recall has been issued for a particular type of equipment. Which patients have been treated with it during the past month?	1. EQUIPMENT → X-RAY 2. X-RAY → RENDERED SERVICE 3. RENDERED SERVICE → ADMITTED PATIENT 4. ADMITTED PATIENT → ACCOUNT 5. ACCOUNT → PATIENT 6. List the patients
	Database management systems have a variety of search and retrieval strategies for optimizing the paths through the database. The syntax for this navigation depends on the query language employed. SQL, for example, would use a series of SELECT and JOIN statements.

physical system must behave according to the data model. For example, if the model indicates that the existence of entity B depends on the existence of entity A, the physical system must prevent creation of record B before the creation of record A. The ability of the system to change is greatest with the relational system, least with stand-alone files.

In this mapping process, the resulting physical structures bear little resemblance to the logical model. Multiple entities frequently are collapsed into single record types. Or, a single entity may be split into multiple physical files. In hierarchical/network systems the logic of the relationships gets lost because the data base segments are connected by physical pointers instead of key fields, which more closely reflect the logic. This is caused by the nature of the DBMS, and also by physical performance: how the user needs to access the data, required speed of access, and so on. If two entities are accessed together frequently, this is a reason to collapse them. This is the case with Account and Admitted Patient, Ordered Service and Rendered Service, and X-ray and Read X-ray.

The situation is further complicated when one has to map the data model to multiple physical systems (as is shown on subsequent pages of this chapter).

Figure 5.27 does not specify the type of data-base management system or the characteristics of the pages and clusters. It just shows that the Patient entity has been mapped directly to a patient file; the Account entity and Admitted Patient entity have been collapsed into the account file; the Image Data attribute of the X-ray entity has been split out into a separate optical disk system for purposes of efficient storage and retrieval; the X-ray, Read X-ray, and X-ray Participant entities have all been collapsed into a single X-ray file.

4.1 Separate "Flat" Files

These files can be difficult to manage because the application programs have the responsibility for enforcing the rules of the data model. For example, you may not insert an account into the data base if you do not have a corresponding patient.

- Account, Admitted Patient, and Consultation are collapsed into one physical Accounts File.
- Ordered Service and Rendered Service are collapsed into one physical Orders File.
- X-ray and X-ray Participant are collaped into one physical X-ray File.
- The X-ray entity is split into a second physical file, the Image File, which contains the binary form of the image.
- The Patient entity is mapped directly into a Patients File. Other entities (such as Physician, Equipment, etc.) are also mapped into their own respective master file.

This collapsing is shown in Figure 5.28.

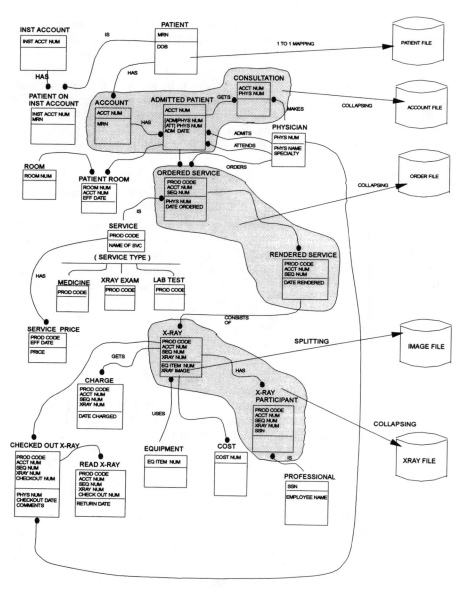

Figure 5.27 Mapping of logical model to physical system.

Account Record: Some systems even collapse the Patient entity into the Accounts File; this situation is frequently found in older hospital information systems. This makes it exceedingly difficult to identify all the accounts that belong to a single patient. It also makes it difficult to

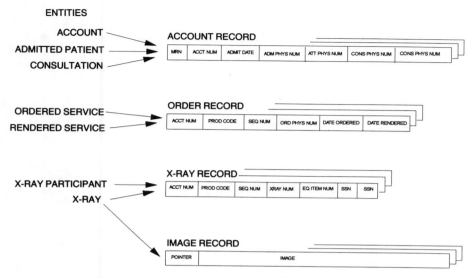

Figure 5.28 Collapsing into a flat file system.

establish a master patient data base. No provision is made for multiple policies; this complicates insurance verification and billing. The guarantor is also collapsed into the patient record; it is therefore not possible to associate the guarantor with the accounts that have been guaranteed. No provision is made for associating multiple visits with an account; a new account has to be opened up for each new visit.

Order Record: This collapsing mostly violates the "no nulls" rule, and is not so harmful to the logic of the model. Other collapsings, which violate the "repeating values" rule, are more harmful.

X-ray Record: While in theory the number of participants may be unlimited, in practice the data base has to be designed to accommodate some specific number; for example, three.

Image Record: In many systems the images themselves are stored on optical disk. The DBMS that manages the structured data about the film has a "pointer" to the image and calls another program to access it on the optical disk.

4.2 Hierarchical/Network DBMS

Figure 5.29 shows a mapping into a hierarchical DBMS, using the segment types identified in the previous section. Hierarchical and network data base management systems use pointers instead of key fields to link segments. This means that, for a given segment, there is no logical indication of its parent segment. If one needs to access the parent, this is done through an upward pointer. While the use of this technology for

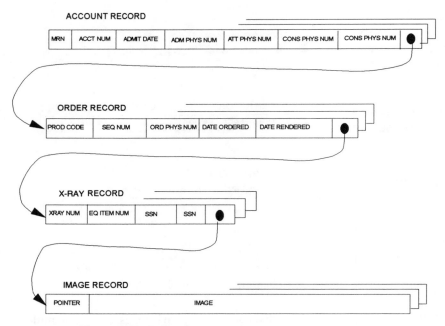

Figure 5.29 Collapsing into a pointer-based system.

new development is declining significantly, many "legacy" systems have been written in it, and they will either have to be converted or linked to newer systems.

In Figure 5.29 an Account-Stay-Patient record is linked to its Order records by a pointer, represented by the arrow. The key for each Account record is the Account Number. The individual Order records are kept in Product Code Sequence. The individual X-ray records are kept in sequence of occurrence.

Several issues arise when the hospital collapses its entities and uses a pointer-based DBMS. First, it is difficult to navigate the data base. Second, over time, it becomes increasingly difficult to understand the logical structure of the data.

In these mappings, the physical data structures must behave according to the logic of the data model. This is the advantage of using a Relational Data Base Management System (RDBMS), which has built-in integrity constraints. This is very difficult with flat files, because they require that all the logic of integrity constraints be placed in the application programs. With pointer-based systems, the logic of the data model is obscured by the physical arrangement of the data base segments, which makes it difficult to combine segments across different hierarchies. To improve understandability, many vendors of pointer-based systems have developed SQL front ends for query activity.

4.3 Relational Data Base Management System

Here the mapping is likely to be more straightforward, with physical indexes into the data base tables. When they first appeared, relational systems were not particularly efficient—their physical storage and access mechanisms were analogous to the logical model, and performance suffered. Over the past ten years relational vendors have been optimizing their systems for speed, and for most applications they are sufficient. Other vendors of non-relational systems have put SQL front ends on their systems, so the data can be accessed and manipulated effectively without knowing the details of the pointer system. However, under the surface these systems are still difficult to restructure.

4.4 Object-Oriented Data Bases

Object-oriented data base management systems appear to address both the logical shortcomings of the relational model and the physical shortcomings of the storage and retrieval mechanisms that underlie them. This will be discussed in greater detail on subsequent pages.

Enterprise Data Model

Ultimately, the hospital will have to construct an Enterprise Data Model. It is called "enterprise" because it spans the hospital, accommodating all the departmental views. This company-wide model is often referred to as the "conceptual schema." This conceptual schema will be mapped into multiple physical systems. In addition to its department-specific entities, the Diagnostic Imaging model contains entities that are found in many departments and many information systems. They include: Patient, Account, Order, Physician, Equipment, Charge, and Cost.

In theory, there are three different approaches to constructing an enterprise model: (1) Do everything at once, top-down, for every area of the hospital; (2) develop the fully attributed key-based data model for each department separately, and try to integrate them afterward; and (3) develop the enterprise model to the key-based level, then work on the models for individual areas and iteratively integrate them into the enterprise model. The first approach is not feasible; it takes too long. The second approach is not feasible because it is too difficult to reconcile data models at the fully attributed level. The third approach is the most reasonable; it steers a middle course. Developing a key-based enterprise model can be done in a reasonable amount of time. The details of key-based models are not so overwhelmingly complex that they prevent integration. The enterprise model is expanded with each departmental model that is done. The departmental model takes the enterprise model as its point of departure and moves to the key-based level. As the department's model changes, the enterprise model is updated to reflect this.

In constructing the enterprise model, one follows the steps outlined in Sections 1 through 3, repeating them for each hospital department. This analysis should be done at organizational levels that correspond roughly to the value chain. Levels such as "Operations" or "Finance" are too general. It should be more specific, such as Admitting, Patient Accounting, Medical Records, Nursing, ICU, Emergency Room, Laboratory, Pharmacy, Research Department, Marketing, and so forth.

The departmental view is defined to the key-based level and then reconciled to the enterprise key-based model. In this process, broader definitions are discovered for departmental entities, and more specific categories are discovered for enterprise entities. New attributes and relationships are frequently added to the enterprise model. In general, the enterprise model will use more N:N relationships than departmental models (because of its greater generality). Many questions of terminology will have to be resolved. Like the English language, a business has "data synonyms" and "data homonyms." An entity may acquire additional attributes and/or relationships, or its meaning may be redefined. Figure 5.30 assumes that an enterprise model has been constructed, and that its first expansion has been to accommodate the Diagnostic Imaging model. Subsequent expansions are slated for Patient Accounting and Lab. It can be seen that Patient Accounting and Lab have common entities such as Patient, Account, Charge, and Physician. Each has its own specific set of entities. The departmental entities cluster together in constellations, with the common entities serving as bridges. Their key attributes are critical to the physical integration of the systems that implement them.

In most hospitals the enterprise model will be implemented with multiple information systems. The data model shows how they fit together logically so that their behavior will fit with the activities of the hospital. When the data resides in physically distinct systems, there are two approaches to providing an integrated view: (1) Employ a report writer that can access and combine data from different systems; (2) extract the data from their native systems and combine them into a single data base. The latter is fairly straightforward, provided that the hospital understands the structure of the data. See Figure 5.31. On the data side, there are two issues that impact the systems' ability to fit the business: access and synchronization. On the network side, there are many other issues, which will be discussed in Chapter 6: Technical Architecture.

Even though every organization has its own unique strategy and structure, within a given industry segment the data models show a lot of commonality. There are significant differences among hospitals in different segments, including their data models. A tertiary-care facility needs to have unlimited Diagnosis and Consulting Physician entities, while a typical adult critical-care facility does not. A chain needs to have a more complicated Organization entity. A facility that provides patient services to other hospitals needs to have an Institutional Account entity. A

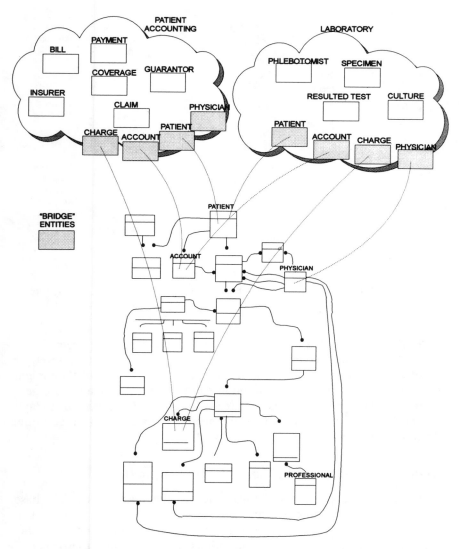

Figure 5.30 Entities common across multiple views of the data.

veteran's hospital does not need the Bill entity, while other hospitals do. A children's hospital requires aliases, since a child may have stepparents over the years. A rural acute-care facility needs only a single consulting physician, while a tertiary-care facility needs many—perhaps a dozen. HMOs do not need the concept of a "Guarantor." A government-run hospital does not need the idea of "Cost."

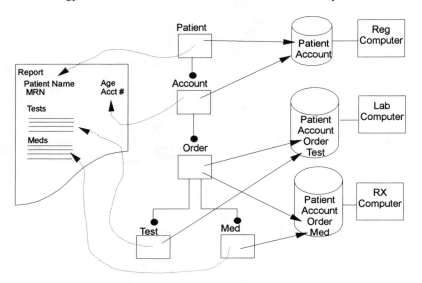

Figure 5.31 Data model mediating between reporting views and file layouts.

A more generic feature, however, is the increased requirement for capturing insurance coverage data. It is important to capture three or more coverages, since husband and wife can both work and they might have supplementary policies. In the model of a previous health care generation, it was enough to know that a patient had insurance. In today's model, for a different generation, one needs to relate the coverage to the diagnosis and treatment for a specific visit.

Synchronization and Ownership of Data Bases

The preceding discussion naturally leads to the question of data base synchronization. If there are multiple data bases, how are they kept in synch? Numerous control issues arise around the common entities. One department "owns" the data, while others use it. Usually, the owner of the data is the department that created it. For example, Business Services owns Account because it creates this entity. The Lab owns Test Result. Problems occur when a user system has its own physical copy of the data. How does the owner ensure that the user department makes the correct synchronization changes (they may not all be automated) and does not make any other changes to the data? How can the owner be sure that the user's system will process this entity as the owner wants (deletion, retention, etc.)?

There are certain business activities, or events, which change the state of an entity (or which create an entity). For example: Admission, Discharge, Order, and Charge all create common entities that must be synchronized across systems. There is a standard for this called HL7. When an event occurs, the owner of that data broadcasts a message to all systems that have an interest in that data (i.e., that have duplicated that data), so that they can change their data bases to reflect this new state of affairs.

Figure 5.32 shows how the admission of a patient triggers the broadcast of a message from the Registration system to the Nursing and Lab systems, containing data relevant to the Patient and the Account. Conversely, when a Charge event occurs in either the Nursing or Lab system, a message is broadcast to the Registration system.

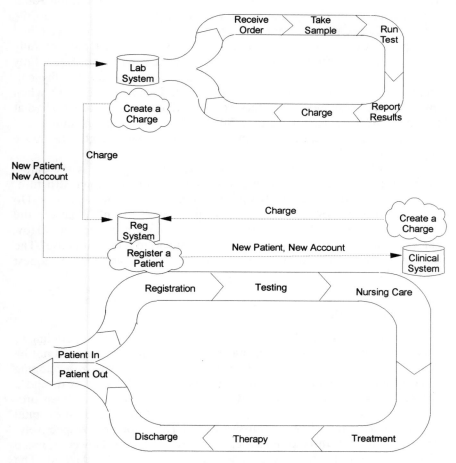

Figure 5.32 Database synchronization triggers.

Other Uses of a Data Model

A data model is a useful tool for many different activities:

1. Systems planning
2. Integration/interfacing
3. Requirements definition/design

One of the most difficult aspects of working in an organization is trying to achieve communication between departments. A requirements definition team will have different backgrounds, and they will deal with many different parties, each with vastly differing views of the world and vocabularies to express these views: ROI/Market Share/Retention Rate/ Practitioner Data Base/Assignment versus Partition/Screen Builder/File Segments/Concentrators. Many efforts to define requirements have failed to capture user requirements properly. The systems staff did not fully understand what they heard. Moreover, the users did not even fully understand what they were saying. When I say something to my collocutor, how do I know that he has understood what I have said? When my collocutor responds, how does he know that I have understood what he has said? One technique to validate that mutual understanding has occurred is to represent the communication through an image. The image is the data model.

Another area where the communication vehicle applies is the Information Center. The Information Center is a new organizational structure. It is an organization that deals with end-user data questions such as: Do you have a report on . . . ? What does this number mean? What are the data sources for . . . ? Which systems have the most accurate data? How can I get access to a system? How can I download to a PC data base? The data model allows the Information Center analyst to map the user request into a solution.

Systems Planning

A hospital intending to develop its own systems can use data modeling to analyze the data that the systems have in common so that they will not be developed in isolation. Assume that a hospital is considering developing three different systems: Telemarketing, a Preferred Patient card, and a Donor Tracking system. Three different systems efforts have been proposed because these activities are performed by three different hospital organizations: Marketing, Admissions, and Development, respectively. As a consequence, three different projects are suggested. However, much of the data is redundant. A common data base could be devised. The data base could be partitioned to allow the systems to be developed in a staged fashion. Its data model would show what data need to be added if the functionality of one of the systems were to be increased to replace the other two.

When a person calls into the hospital, s/he is identified as either a donor, sales lead, or program member (cardholder, for example). While each system has its specific functionality, each also contains common functionality (enforced by the Data Model) for initial contact activity and follow-up activity. In this way, the hospital can obtain an integrated view of its contacts with the outside world.

Data Modeling in Integration and Interfacing

For a more detailed discussion, see Chapter 6: Technical Architecture, where we discuss the HL7 and MEDIX committee efforts to define standard transactions that can be used to synchronize heterogeneous data bases.

The term "legacy system" refers to those older systems that are particularly important for operations, and which cannot be replaced easily. Systems integration requires that a strategy be developed for accommodating these systems. The term "accommodate" is used because integrating these systems is most difficult. In any case, one must understand their logic to deal with them. First, they are poorly documented, and this interferes with data modeling. Second, when the systems are based on flat files most of the semantics of the data model is contained in the programs themselves, and thus is difficult to model.

Requirements Definition and System Design

In requirements definition projects, most time and effort are invested in defining what functions are needed (process bias), and little attention is paid to an orderly analysis and presentation of the data requirements. The data requirements, in turn, impact the functional requirements—if one has the inappropriate data structure in the data base, certain pieces of functionality will never be achieved, without major restructuring of data and programs. A very effective technique for evaluating a vendor during a demonstration is to construct scenarios and have the vendor show how her/his system can perform the scenario. The data model can help to structure these scenarios. Scenario 1: "Show me how to get a list of all the patient's past accounts while I am setting up a new account," Scenario 2: "Show me how to display all outstanding orders while I am creating a new order." Trying to follow this logic on computer screens alone will distract the hospital from understanding the true functionality of the system.

Another weakness of traditional requirements definition is in specifying reporting requirements. Page after page is written specifying what fields are needed, how they should be sorted, and so forth. No one is ever satisfied with it, and it is never exhaustive. The data model encompasses all the entities and relationships used to generate the reporting requirements. By concentrating on the query software and the vendor's match to the hospital's data model, one can walk through the model with the vendor, and s/he can show selected paths through the model.

Policy Definition

Frequently, information systems are blamed for the hospital's failure to enforce policies. There is some validity to this claim. Underlying the Business Architecture is a series of policies and procedures. Many of these policies are captured in the Data Model. For example, a Patient should have only one Medical Record Number; there must be a valid Account before a Charge can be issued. If the information system is implemented in conformance with the data model, then the DBMS enforces these policy constraints. In this way, the information systems are aligned with the business architecture. As discussed previously, policies frequently change when the industry experiences a paradigm shift or when a hospital embarks on a new strategy.

It can be shown that many of the these breakdowns in the value chain represent policy violations (see Table 5.7). For example, the hospital has a policy that each patient should receive one and only one Medical Record Number, for purposes of identification. This policy could be violated either procedurally, technically, or through data policy. Other chapters address the procedural and technical aspects of this.

Hospitals can have very specific policies such as "If the child is less than two years old, the Attending Physician must be a pediatrician." There is a debate about how much "semantics" to embed in the model and enforce with the DBMS. A simple example of this is the registration process, in which the admitting privileges of the physician must be verified, the creditworthiness of the guarantor must be verified, and the last visit must be checked. The hospital needs to set up institutional data policies, which can be understood by both general management and technical management.

Miscellaneous Issues

There are two important issues: data structure and data modality. So far, this book has dealt with traditional "structured" data and classical relational data models. Structured data is traditional "data processing" data. Each record type and field has a rigid structure: Medical Record Number, Patient Name, and so on. If there is text in fields, it is quite limited. Relational theory was developed when computers were capable of pro-

Table 5.7 Data Policies and Their Violation

Area	Value detractor	Violated policy
Registration	The same patient gets registered with different medical record numbers because there are multiple registration systems—one for IP, another for OP.	A patient has one, and only one, Medical Record Number. For a given encounter, a patient has an account, which may be either an inpatient or outpatient account type [but an account is still an account].
Clinical management	It is difficult to obtain a horizontally integrated picture of the patient's treatment for a given stay: lab tests, medicines, treatments progress notes. It is difficult to obtain a longitudinally integrated picture of the patient, for diagnosis purposes.	A patient has a stay. This stay has orders, and the orders may be for tests, medications, or treatments. A stay requires progress notes. A patient may have multiple stays, over time.
Billing	There is a separate system for collections. Data is not received from the collection system, and creditworthiness is not accurately reflected at the time of admission. Bills go to the wrong addresses when the demographic data is in the Registration system, but is not updated in the Billing system.	An account may become a collection account, but a collection account is still an account [and its status should be available when reviewing other types of accounts]. A patient receives an account for a stay. This account has a mailing address to which the bill should be sent. [There is not a Registration account separate from a Billing account]

cessing only traditional data processing data. However, there are other kinds of data: lengthy, unstructured text, which contains most of our knowledge about patients (i.e., physician notes in the patient chart); voice; still images, cinematic images, and wave forms. Improvements in technology (CD ROM and networks) and methodology (object modeling) permit the capture and manipulation of these different data types as though they are part of a single data base.

Data Bases versus Knowledge Bases

Future data models will have to deal with knowledge bases. Traditional data models and data bases deal with "descriptive" data—the data base presents the data as it *was* or *is*. There is a growing body of literature on "knowledge bases." A knowledge base is a special kind of data base that contains the facts and rules that a human expert uses in the performance of his job. (A physician, for example, is an expert on physiology and diseases.) The rules can be weighted with probabilities. For example, when a doctor examines a patient, the doctor knows that a given set of symptoms in 90 percent of the cases indicates a particular disease. Table 5.8 compares what the physician knows about a particular patient versus what s/he knows about the disease and patients in general.

Knowledge bases do not contain descriptive data, but rather generalizations and prescriptive or normative material. The models that underlie them differ by their prescriptiveness and generality, as summarized in Table 5.9. There are many ways to represent knowledge: as decision trees, as rules, as semantic networks, and as tables (entities). Semantic networks are very similar to data models. The extensive use of subcategories in a data model helps with knowledge representation. The term "frame" is similar to "entity." It is important to note that the *representation* of knowledge is different from the *programming* techniques that implement it on a computer.[2]

Table 5.8 Descriptive Data vs. Prescriptive Data

Descriptive data	Prescriptive/probabilistic data
"John Smith, Jr., *was* born prematurely, at 28 weeks. He had been transferred to the hospital. He *was* in respiratory distress, at risk for sepsis, *had* feeding problems because of an immature digestive system, and *had* thermal regulation problems due to low body weight. This *was* followed by a series of treatments that consisted of keeping John in an oxygen tent and warmer, checking for an elevated white blood count, and intravenous feeding."	"A child who is born at 28 weeks most likely *will* have respiratory distress, risk of sepsis, and feeding problems. This child *should* receive the following treatments: oxygen tent and warmer, WBC tests, and intravenous feeding."
The model and data base represent the facts as they are, not as they should be.	The "knowledge base" portion of this model grows as medical research grows. The above entities could be expanded to include potential complications. New entities are added, frequently arising from the attributes of the descriptive model.

---

[2] For a comprehensive, traditional treatment of the nature of medical data, see Marsden S. Blois, *Information and Medicine: The Nature of Medical Descriptions*, Berkeley and Los Angeles: University of California Press, 1984.

Table 5.9 Differences between Data Bases and Knowledge Bases

Data base	Knowledge base
Deals with individuals. Contains the record for a patient identified as MRN 98647.	Generalized; that is, it does not deal with individual cases. In a sense, it could be considered summarized data—knowledge summarized from a large experience base.
Descriptive. Describes how things are or were. The patient had diagnosis of hypertension.	Predictive or "normative." It specifies what *should* be done, not what has already been done.
Things are either yes or no. A patient either has a characteristic or he does not.	Often has probabilities attached to its entities. Attributes can have "approximate" values.

Figure 5.33 illustrates the difference between a data model and a knowledge model. The entities outside of the shaded area represent the Data Model underlying the *data base*, which holds the actual Diagnoses, Problems, and Treatments for given Patients. The entities within the shaded area represent the model that underlies the *knowledge base*. It has nothing to say about individually identifiable patients.

Object Modeling and Object-Oriented DBMS

In recent years, "object-oriented" analysis and programming tools have become very popular, and its advocates claim that object-oriented Data Base Management Systems will make relational data bases obsolete. It is important to distinguish between modeling techniques and programming/implementation techniques. The differences in analytic techniques are not large when one compares E-R models with object models. It is true that object-oriented programming has great advantages in terms of productivity and understandability. (See Table 5.10.) Eventually, relational DBMS's will be extended to embrace many of the OODBMS features, and the OODBMS will be changed to incorporate some of the integrity constraints of the relational systems. Ultimately, they may merge.

Clinical Data Models

Clinical data models are models of physiological data, as opposed to administrative data, but their entities are still part of the enterprise model. Clinical data is quite different than administrative data for several reasons: (1) It is much more complex (e.g., text, images, wave forms) and there are many more relationships to manage; (2) much clinical data is unstructured text; (3) the nature of the data is still being discovered—researchers constantly learn more about the side effects of drugs, for

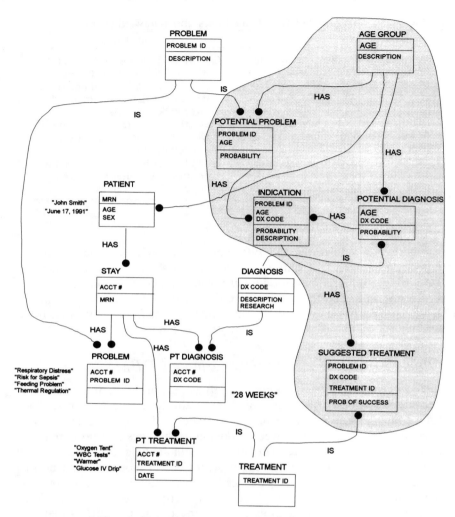

Figure 5.33 Data model versus knowledge model.

instance (on the other hand, except for new regulatory requirements, there is nothing new about a patient bill); (4) it is closely linked to knowledge bases. Clinical data bases are probably best implemented in object technology. Object implementations appear to work better for models with large numbers of tables and complex nested components, such as a bill of materials. Indeed, the human body can be viewed as one large Bill of Materials. The data produced by the human body during one 24-hour stay in the hospital overwhelms the amount of administrative

Table 5.10 Relational Technology vs. Object-Oriented Technology

Relational technology	Object world
Handles less complex transactions, such as registering a patient.	Handles more complex transactions, such as manipulating an architectural drawing, or patient chart.
Incorporates relatively little explicit semantics.	Incorporates more application semantics.
Inefficiently handles arrays and repeating groups.	Handles time series and arrays more efficiently.
Does not easily accommodate data types such as unstructured text, pictures, and voice.	Easily accommodates complex data types.
Has built-in integrity constraints.	Has no formal mechanism for specifying integrity constraints.
Mathematically provable.	Not mathematically provable.
Data is independent of the programs that manipulate it.	Data may contain the program ("method") that acts upon it.

data produced for that same patient for the same period. Object-oriented data bases also appear to work better with data types like drawings and voice. Relational implementations work well for highly structured business data.

6
Technical Architecture

GENERAL DISCUSSION

The Business Architecture defines the structure of the business processes and their alignment with hospital strategy. It is supported by the Data Architecture, which specifies how the business fits together logically so that the data can be used to manage the hospital in a strategic and integrated fashion. This data, however, has to be collected and distributed to the business processes. The framework in which this is done is called the Technical Architecture. Computer networks distribute data to the hospital's business processes, and the Technical Architecture specifies how these networks should "fit" with these business processes: Can they fit with the decentralization, coordination, and sequencing of the business processes?

Fit with the Business Process

Under the influence of Total Quality Management principles, many companies have started to reengineer their business processes. Networking advances provide even greater possibilities for support of the value chain. They can overcome value detractors caused by distance, time lags, lack of coordination, and data gaps, allowing activities to be tightly integrated and crisply executed.

Historically, however, computers, while they facilitated some business processes, introduced lags and inconsistencies into other business processes. This can be illustrated in the following hypothetical case, where the Technical Architecture does not fit with the Business and Data Architectures. There exist two comparable hospitals, both urban adult acute-care hospitals with similar services and patient populations. They have equivalent levels of organizational structure and business processes.

They both have well-defined policies and procedures, with appropriately trained staff, and efficient work flows. Both hospitals have a multi-vendor information system consisting of three major modules with broadly equivalent functionality: Pharmacy, Laboratory, and Registration/Patient Accounting. Hospital A, however, has installed them as stand-alone systems, while hospital B has them attached to a common backbone network and they exchange data with each other.

Despite its operational efficiencies, hospital A is at a disadvantage relative to hospital B. While each of its systems has excellent functionality, they are stand-alone, not connected to any other system for purposes of data synchronization and access, and thus the overall business cycle suffers. This is a classic case of suboptimization. Some of the impacts on the ability to compete in time and with quality are the following:

- In order to avoid duplicate data entry, tapes are used for data exchange. Patient Demographic changes go from the HIS to the ancillaries, and the ancillaries send charges to the HIS. The tapes are exchanged at midnight, and so the information systems are out of synch with the business processes.
- While the systems facilitate an individual department's activity, they prevent the smooth flow of operations among departments and across the enterprise. The whole is less than the sum of its parts.
- The lab results cannot easily be interpreted because the medications are not known. Two terminals are needed.
- Charges are batched, with a delay of twenty-four to forty-eight hours, preventing production of a "demand bill."
- Teaching and research functions do not have an integrated view of the patient—either horizontally or vertically.
- Extra manual effort is expended to avoid duplication of Medical Record Numbers or inaccuracies in patient data caused by redundant, unsynchronized data bases.
- Complete and accurate diagnosis is hampered by lack of access to previous visits.
- The Billing data base is not connected to the Collection data base, causing staff to use two terminals.

Figure 6.1 illustrates the concept of misalignment between Technical Architecture and Business/Data Architecture. Stand-alone systems cannot fit the smooth flow of operations and integrated structure of the data (of course, not all hospitals have an effective Business Architecture). Information technology may facilitate local service, but it also creates systemic "service discontinuities" and "wait states" across departments, as shown in Figure 6.2, in an era when patient service and fast response are paramount. Information systems should support the interactions

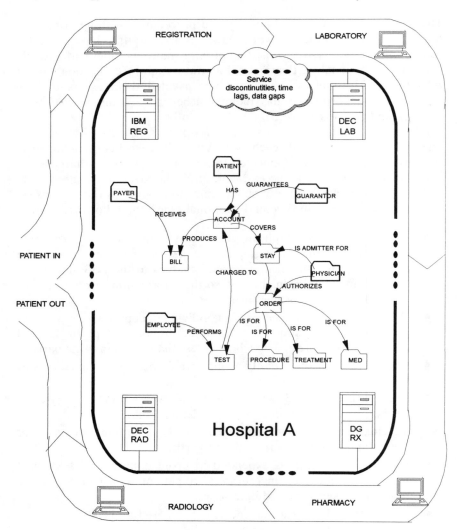

Figure 6.1 Misalignment of architectures.

among the departmental value chains. Instead, they distract from the core business tasks. Each departmental system in Figure 6.1 has its own stand-alone network, isolated from other departmental systems. This discontinuity is shown by dotted lines between systems.

Contrast this situation with hospital B, which has designed its systems to fit with the business processes (Figure 6.3). This hospital has installed a backbone network, and all work travels over it. Each major information system is synchronized with all the others, in real time, as the patient

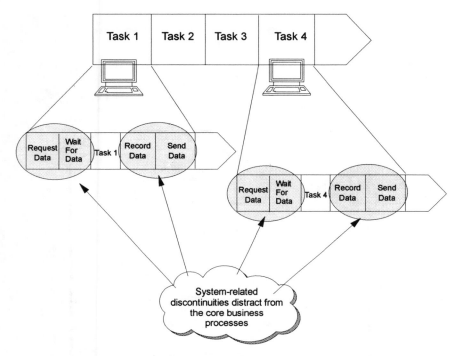

Figure 6.2 Non-essential tasks imposed by misaligned systems.

passes through the hospital from department to department. Every user has a single workstation that provides a window into the information resources of the hospital. The benefits: Clinicians obtain an integrated view of the patient for a given stay, as well as longitudinally; Billing knows about a service provided as soon as it is rendered; everybody is informed of schedule changes; lab technicians have access to Pharmacy's data base. The end result: tighter integration, better service, higher accuracy.

There is a third possibility: hospital C has all these departmental modules as one integrated system from a single vendor. This system may sacrifice some functionality, but it provides a better fit with the departmental work flows and it has all the data stored together. (This is the theory—in reality, many single-vendor solutions are far from integrated.) This represents the long-standing debate: Is it better to have a single-vendor system with "adequate" functionality and integration, or a stand-alone system with rich functionality but no inherent integration? Historically, single-vendor solutions have been more appropriate for smaller hospitals, which can tolerate the more "shallow" functionality. Any vendor that proposed to have a comprehensive system (Billing, Registration, Medical Records, Ancillaries, and Nursing) had to sacrifice

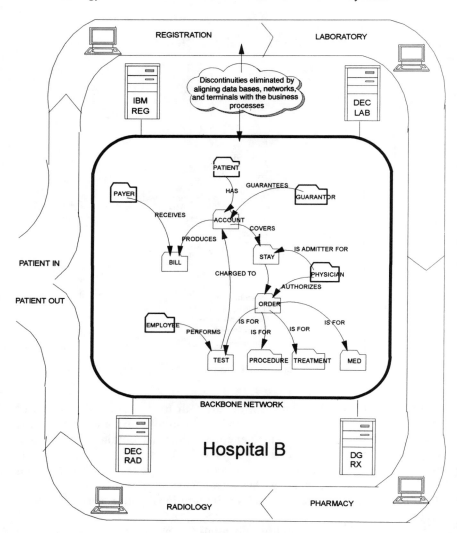

Figure 6.3 Alignment of architectures.

functionality. On the other hand, a vendor that provided a "niche" application with rich functionality (e.g., stand-alone Medical Records) by definition could not provide integration. This trade-off is illustrated in Figure 6.4. As mentioned, there have been some single-vendor solutions that were not integrated, and which placed the user in the "low-low" cell.

Recently, this conventional wisdom has been challenged by both vendors and individual hospitals. Because of advances in networks, data bases, and the standards for linking them, it is becoming possible to achieve the unattainable "high-high" quadrant. A hospital can purchase

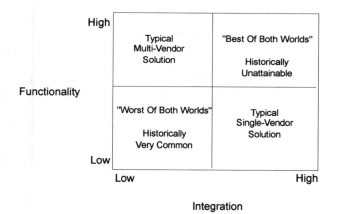

Figure 6.4 Trade-off of functionality versus integration.

stand-alone modules and "integrate" them by connecting them to a common network and making them exchange data. This provides both the breadth and depth of functionality.

Technology Evolution

One may examine the general evolution of Information Technology under this rubric of functionality and integration, since there are two major ways in which technology supports the value chain: by facilitating and blending in with a single activity, and by connecting multiple activities. The term "functionality" refers not just to traditional functionality, but also to transparency and ease of use, the degree to which technology intrudes upon the business activity:

- Does the system force the user to perform numerous manual steps to make up for gaps in the software?
- Does the user have to do a manual lookup of data not accommodated by the system?
- Is there a twenty-four hour wait for the system to process the data that the user has entered?
- Does the user spend more time trying to understand the computer than dealing with the patient?
- Is the system accessible whenever the user needs it?

Over time, computer systems have increasingly merged with the operations they support. Transparency is particularly important when a hospital employs multiple systems. The designs of these systems can be quite different. One system requires that the user select items from a menu; another forces the users to remember commands; a third might be graphically oriented and require the user to make selections with a mouse. The ways of getting on-line help and looking up codes in master tables may be different. The same printer might have different names.

If I place an order through one computer, I may get some rudimentary statuses and results back from the Lab system, but I will never get the richness and functionality of the Lab system duplicated in the Orders system. Therefore, in order to obtain the most data on a series of Lab tests, I must use the Lab computer. "Integration" refers to the synchronization of data across many computer systems, systems interoperability, and the use of resources on other computers:

- Do I have to enter data into multiple computers?
- When I enter data into one computer, do I have to wait one to two days before it is reflected in other systems?
- If the data is subsequently changed in one system, will it be reflected in the other systems?

As information systems have evolved from mainframes through PCs and Local Area Networks, both functionality and integration have steadily increased, as portrayed in Figure 6.5, which shows the evolution from IBM 360/370 mainframes (circa 1965) up through the early 1990s.

Mainframes: Initially, there was no possibility of "integrating" computers with the Business Architecture. They were enormous, expensive machines. They were operated centrally, remote from the operations of the hospital. Jobs supporting business activities were batched and run after hours. The computers were stand-alone. Few end users had access to the computer; they had arcane commands; initially, they employed only teletype terminals for access. With a few notable exceptions, they were used for back-office applications, where integration with the business process was not required. Typical applications were billing, payroll and general ledger. Although these processes are not part of the core value chain, their automation obviously provided value. It displaced much manual labor, providing greater speed and accuracy.

Minicomputers: Provided an improvement in functionality. They were somewhat more aligned with the Business Architecture of individual departments inasmuch as they could be placed locally, within a building or user department. In general, there was little connectivity among them, particularly if they came from different vendors, so there was no real improvement in integration across the hospital. Data was still incompatible and/or inaccessible. The user had to employ multiple terminals. Each minicomputer vendor had his own type of terminal, and they differed in many respects: the number of lines they could display, the highlighting,

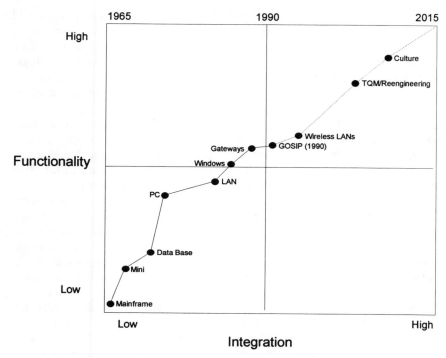

Figure 6.5 Evolution of information technology.

the functions performed by each key, how it processed the data, and so forth.

Much hospital work has the nature of a job shop (Lab, Pharmacy, etc.); such a departmental orientation is well suited for minicomputers. The hospital as a whole did not benefit because the data was not synchronized among systems, but competitive environments at that time did not require this. This is in contrast to airlines and banks, whose structures and competitive environments depended on mainframes for centralized processing of large volumes of transactions across a wide geographcial area. Each minicomputer vendor developed his own conventions for networking.

Data Base Management Systems: Increased both functionality and integration by providing the capability to manage data across departments. The increase in functionality was greater than that of integration because these data bases did not integrate data across systems and departments. For example, Lab files became organized, but could not be combined with Pharmacy files.

Personal Computers: Signaled a revolution in functionality, and this laid the groundwork for increased integration. The end user had a full computer located on the desk top or lab bench, and this computer could support many more business processes than a dumb terminal. Some areas of transparency were not affected; each application still had its own look and feel. But at least each application was now accessible through a single terminal—because the employee had a full computer, he could use its power to "emulate" or imitate the various "dumb" terminals required by the multiple systems, if his job required it.

LANs: Local Area Networks greatly advanced integration. When they were first introduced, however, their primary use was for small work groups to share printers and do simple electronic mail and file sharing. Over time they have evolved to include sophisticated multi-user data bases, group text retrieval, and common calendaring, resulting in the linking of whole departments and even companies. Lately, LANs have been extended to include internetworking, mainframe links, and greater numbers of users. Although LANs provide the potential for integration, the applications that run on them have to be designed for integration. They have to be multi-user, data-base-oriented, and Email enabled. These issues are still being resolved. Furthermore, the LANs themselves must be designed for interoperability. They must allow the user to move from LAN to LAN in a transparent fashion, according to the dictates of his business process. Currently, this is not widely feasible.

Windows: The release of Microsoft Windows 3.0 was another milestone in the evolution of technology. This software makes it possible for all PC applications to have the same look and feel, increasing functionality. It also makes it possible for applications to share data more easily, and so it increases integration. Any software program that runs with Windows must conform to certain programming standards, and this ensures that they will have a high degree of interoperability with other programs.

Gateways: This is a generic term for such devices as "bridges," "routers," and "gateways" (each of which has a very specific meaning in the world of networking). These are hardware devices that allow the extension and interconnection of networks. They can connect the same type of network, or "translate" from one network to another as they connect them. This represents a major step toward integration. Once again, gateways can connect multiple networks, but the end-user applications must be designed to interact and take advantage of these gateways.

GOSIP: This book has selected a regulatory event, rather than a hardware/software milestone, to mark the transition from lower to higher levels of integration. "GOSIP" stands for "Government OSI Profile." In the late 1980s the U.S. government announced that, starting in August 1990, its systems vendors had to make their systems compatible with the Open Systems Interconnect (OSI) model (to the extent that it is complete). The period 1987–1990 witnessed enormous growth in standards-setting activities for "open systems." Many vendors formed consortiums to develop standards for networking. The Open Software Foundation was created. Many governmental agencies (state and federal) saw the value of purchasing "open" systems. However, most agencies viewed this from a cost perspective rather than a service perspective.

The OSI is a model for how systems should be designed so that they may be aligned with the business processes. OSI is discussed in greater detail in this chapter. Most OSI documents are not written for the general manager. They define protocols for how systems should interact, with regard to such things as Email, file access and transfer, terminal emulation, and internetworking.

Wireless LANs: The potential for integration surged ahead when wireless LANs were introduced. These are Local Area Networks that allow connection through radio waves or infrared waves, eliminating the need for recabling when a user moves his workstation.

Total Quality Management and Business Reengineering: The founding of the Malcolm Baldridge Award for quality management was an important event in American industry. It indicates an important trend to place more emphasis on solving the problems within business processes, rather than simply assigning more resources to their existing structure. This set of values and methodology has started to spread into the area of Information Systems. The belief is that it is wrong to automate a manual process without making redesign of the process a fundamental part of the automation activity. This marks an important milestone. No longer will advances in functionality and integration be achieved through technology alone. They now will be led by advances in methods and an emphasis on standards.

Culture: It took approximately twenty-five years to reach a moderate level of "fit" between the Technical Architecture and the Business Architecture (from mainframes to gateways). The next twenty-five years will be spent in elaborating the standards and perfecting the tools and techniques. However, during this period, the greatest challenge, and the highest level of activity, will be in changing the culture of U.S. companies. This is part of the paradigm shift required by TQM. Ever since the rise of large hierarchical corporations in the nineteenth century, U.S. companies have been operating in a departmental, conflict-oriented mode. The culture and skill-set of management and employees must be changed, together with the systems for evaluating and rewarding performance. Ultimately, integration of technology with the business process will require that U.S. companies, including hospitals, do things differently. Increasingly, the ability to assimilate integrating technology will depend on the organization's ability to learn (methodology) and its willingness to learn (culture). Winning hospitals will learn faster. This is further proof that the ultimate strategic advantage is the ability of an organization to learn and adapt. And this means that the ultimate strategic asset is the organization's human resources.

Figure 6.5 represents only the theoretical increases in functionality and integration. The gains actually achieved by a given hospital depend on the culture of the organization and the skills of its people. Some hospitals have been able to "squeeze" higher levels of functionality out of a given stage of technology by effective use of policies and procedures. Other hospitals have not been able to achieve the anticipated levels of functionality and integration from a higher stage of technology; they have not had effective policies and procedures. These are issues of Control Architecture, and are discussed in Chapter 7.

Of course, many other technologies have contributed to functionality. This would include mouses, light pens, touch screens, faxes, voice recognition, laser printers, and so forth. Finally, it should also be pointed out that, over time, each technology has shown gains in both functionality and integration (because the technology was enhanced, its methdology was improved, or because the technology was combined with another technology). For example, both the functionality and integration of mainframes have been increased by successive improvements, such as the replacement of teletype machines by CRTs, the replacement of CRTs by PCs running emulation software, the introduction of networking, and the use of data base software.

Business Processes and Standards

In Figure 6.5 the movement of the development line is driven by a combination of technology innovation and standards-based activity. Innovation precedes standards. Innovation within a department or area can "suboptimize" the whole enterprise. A new piece of software or hardware tries to optimize the functionality for its respective department, but it can create service discontinuities across the enterprise. A department's electronic mail system may facilitate patient flow within the department, but not across departments; its integrated data base may help the department, but conflict with the data bases of other departments. In the first half of Figure 6.5 standards played catch-up with innovation. In the second half, standards have come into their own. The more recent milestones are all standards-oriented: GOSIP, TQM, and Culture.

Figure 6.5 shows an increasing alignment of technology with the business process. In terms of physical location, systems have moved from the remote back office to the department, from the department to the desk top, and, finally, from the desk top to any arbitrary location (through hand-held computers and wireless networks). In terms of organization, systems have moved from the enterprise to the department, and from the department to the individual. They are now poised to support work groups and the integrated enterprise.

Because of this growing proximity and ubiquity of technology, general managers must become more involved in its management. However, rather than jump straight into the technical details of information systems, the general manager must approach them from the perspective of the business cycle, asking, "What are the integrating activities of the organization?" This obviously includes alerting all interested parties of any changes in the patient's status, ensuring that all parties are working with the same data, and providing all necessary data to all parties in time to do their jobs. The related systems features are electronic mail, file sharing, data base synchronization, and common access through a single terminal (see Table 6.1). Chapter 4 discussed the use of horizontal organizational structures to prevent service discontinuities; these organizations need systems that are aligned with their activities.

HL7

Health Level Seven is the most familiar standard for health care systems integration. It deals with synchronizing the data in different computers, specifying the structure and contents of the messages that computers must exchange in order to ensure that a change to Patient data will be reflected in every system that contains Patient data. Common data includes ADT data, orders, results, and billing data. Does the patient have the same Medical Record Number in all data bases? Does every data base have the current Patient Name and Address? Is a canceled order reflected in every data base? The technical section of this chapter contains a more detailed discussion.

HL7 will eventually eliminate the need for complex custom interfaces among systems. Many large HIS vendors originally adopted an adversarial stance with regard to HL7, claiming that their existing interfaces were sufficient. This is not surprising, since a generic standard for data exchange represents the risk of lost business because it allows customers to mix and match modules more easily. For this reason, most of the initial proponents of HL7 were smaller vendors, and sellers of niche products. By the nature of their business, they are forced to maintain many interfaces with larger vendors, which are naturally reluctant to open up their systems. The vendors opposed to HL7 do have one valid caveat about HL7. To the extent that a hospital employs systems from multiple vendors, it has to do more management of the relationships among the system components. If a hospital purchases a total system from a single vendor, then the burden is on the vendor to manage the integration of the multiple components.

MEDIX

MEDIX is another standard for the synchronization of data bases. MEDIX is the health care standards subcommittee of the ISO (International

Table 6.1 Connectivity Standards to Support Organizational Integrating Activities

User activity	Integrating activities	Required standards for Information Systems
Registration	The registration clerk needs to be able to inform the Lab Technician and Pharmacist of new patients and changes to patient demographic data.	*Naming*: There should be a standard for referring to all the users of information systems, and for routing a message across the network to these users. For example, if Registration needs to notify Billing of a new Patient, then there should be a convention for determining the path through the network.
Fill prescription	The Pharmacist needs to know medications and allergic reactions the patient has had previously.	*Electronic Mail*: If two systems need to send messages among system users, a standard allows the messages to get from one system to another in a meaningful form.
Result a lab test	The Lab Technician, in order to properly interpret test results, needs to know what meds the patient is taking.	*File Exchange and Access*: An employee should be able to look up all relevant patient information from any system and transfer it to his system.
		Data Base Synchronization: If two systems have a Doctor master file, when a new physician is added to the first system, there should be a standard for communicating that change to the second system, so that it can update its own data base.
		User Interface: If a hospital employee has to use two or more systems in the performance of his job function (e.g., both a Registration and a Scheduling system), there should be a standard for how the user interacts with the systems. There should be a convention for how he opens a file, stores a record, prints a report, etc. There should be a single terminal.
		Document Exchange: The network should allow an employee to combine all the forms of a patient's data and send it to all interested parties. This data includes free-form text, numerical data, images, wave forms, voice recordings, etc.

Standards Organization). MEDIX, however, goes beyond the scope of HL7, including all aspects of connectivity, such as electronic mail, universal addressing, file exchange and access, as well as more technical aspects. While both committees have been in existence for approximately the same period of time, HL7 has managed to publish implementable specifications, while MEDIX is still defining its theoretical framework. There are plans to merge the two, with MEDIX subsuming HL7.

HL7 and MEDIX represent the broader phenomenon of EDI (Electronic Data Interchange). Whether it is used to integrate the systems in one company, or across several companies, EDI ensures that the computer architecture more closely follows the business architecture. EDI is used heavily in banking and manufacturing. Its potential for health care is enormous.

Vendor and User Consortiums

Recently, large groups of influential vendors, sensing that the future is in standards, have come together to accelerate the development of standards based on existing vendor products. There are several emerging standards for transparency. The most prominent one is the Open Software Foundation's "Distributed Computing Environment." The problem with consortiums, however, is that they are subject to manipulation by vendors driven by self-interest and short-term gains. Already one consortium, announced with great fanfare, has been disbanded. This is the Advanced Computing Environment. Some vendors have made "standards-based" computing their strategy.

Levels of Standards

General managers are confronted with a mind-numbing array of technical terms when dealing with network "standards." When discussing their IBM system, they hear: "VSAM, EBCDIC, SNA, SDLC, COAX, SAA, CONTROLLER, HOST." Their DEC system has its own vocabulary: "RDB, ASCII, DNA, ASYNCH, PATHWORKS, TERMINAL SERVER, LAT." The Local Area Network has its own Tower of Babel: "FILE SERVER, ARCNET, ACTIVE HUB, BTRIEVE, IPX." All these terms represent the vendors' terminology for their connectivity conventions. If a general manager tries to deal with vendors on their terms, s/he will be at a disadvantage. The manager must first develop a conceptual framework that allows him or her to evaluate what the vendors are saying. This framework focuses on the Business Architecture and Data Architecture. Figure 6.6 provides such a framework.

From this point of view, a network has three general levels of connectivity. At the first level, does the system in question "plug into" the general network? If not, can this be achieved through conversion and translation? At the second level, can a user of that system be routed over the network? At the third level, what useful interaction can I achieve across this network? Can I exchange electronic mail? Can I access another system's data and combine it with mine? Can I update all data bases with

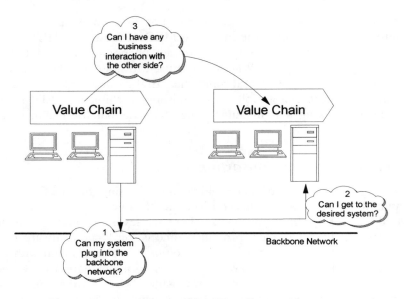

Figure 6.6 Conceptual framework for general managers.

a single transaction? Can I access programs on someone else's system, and will they look like my system? Figure 6.6 illustrates these distinct levels of connectivity. In more concrete terms, a researcher sitting on the Novell network needs to do three things: (1) get on the backbone network; (2) travel across the backbone to other information systems of interest (Registration/Medical Records and Laboratory); (3) once the researcher gets to these other systems, s/he needs to be able to do some productive work: to access data on past visits, diagnoses, and treatments; as well as to access current patients and their lab results, and combine this information with the research on the Novell system.

At each of these levels there are different types of standards.

Level 1: Physical Connection

This is the most basic level of connectivity. Can the hospital plug a given information system into its existing network? Does the system have the same electromechanical characteristics and protocols for data transmission? If not, is there a way to convert them? If the system cannot directly connect, can it connect through a telephone? At this level, decisions are made about the types of cabling that will be used, how it will be laid out, how the network will be segmented, what the protocols will be for controlling access to the network, and so forth. Terms such as Ethernet, Token Ring, Arcnet, Asynch, twisted pair, coaxial cable, wiring closets, hubs, and so on, are at this level. The general manager should not be concerned with these technical issues. However, in many cases, the answers to these technical questions will depend on the characteristics of the Business Architecture (business processes, how they interact, when they interact, with what volumes?), and the general manager must be prepared to define the requirements of the Business Architecture to the technical staff.

Level 2: Routing

After a system is connected to the backbone network, can a user be routed from her/his system across the network to the desired destination? Figure 6.6 presents a simplified model. In reality, there may be several intervening networks between the two systems, and unless the user can get across these networks, there can be no meaningful business interaction between the two systems. For reasons of administration and performance, many users will be isolated on subnetworks, but will still have occasion to travel across the backbone to cooperate with other users. For example, there has been a proliferation of LANs that support departmental functions such as Medical Records coding, Quality Assurance, Risk Management, Human Resources, and Physician Management. Staff in these departments spend most of their time with internal communications, but also have "integrating" needs such as the requirement to synchronize data bases or share Email. For example, each one of the above-mentioned systems has the entity "Physician;" however, Physician Management (Medical Staff Services) is responsible for the creation and change of Physician data, and needs to broadcast these changes to all interested systems. Will all the messages get to the target in their proper sequence? Will demographic updates get to their addressees? Can the lab user get over to the orders machine to check for meds?

Level 3: User Functionality

The general manager should not be concerned with the lower levels, except for definition of Business Architecture requirements. If the system can support the functionality at this third level, then the lower-level components will take care of themselves. This is the level at which meaningful interaction occurs among business processes. This level cannot exist until the two lower levels are in place. It is at this level that the vocabulary of technology and the vocabulary of business begin to converge. The terms "Email protocols" or "data base access protocols" are conceptually obvious to general managers, even though they do not understand the mechanics. This level allows the exchange of electronic mail alerting staff about a patient's condition; can a researcher develop a comprehensive study using data retrieved from the registration, lab, and pharmacy systems? Once the user reaches the desired destination, can s/he do any useful work with or on the other system? Can the user's application "talk" to the other application? Can they exchange files? Can the user send electronic mail to someone on another computer system? Do the applications exchange standard transactions to keep their respective master files synchronized? End-user functionality has great relevance to the health care executive, who expects information sources to be accessible and kept in synch. Can a programmer use a common access method to extract the data from the data bases to build an integrated picture of the patient, for purposes of developing clinical protocols? This is the level at which the protocols for exchanging compound documents (text, numbers, charts, pictures) will be defined, allowing creation of an all-electronic medical record.

Within the business processes there are different types of users, each with different connectivity requirements:

1. "Heads-down" users: Users of a single system, most frequently one that does heavy transaction processing, such as registration or order entry. They need their data base to be synchronized with other data bases. Occasionally, they need to do a lookup in another system. They also need electronic mail, to flag exceptions for other staff.

2. "Data-driven" users: Researchers, analysts, planners, auditors, and diagnosticians. These staff need access to data from a wide variety of systems. They need a lot of data, as opposed to "heads-down" users, who typically work with one record at a time. And they need a lot of tools to manipulate the data.

3. "General" users: These are most likely managers who need integration for communications such as Email, for occasional "data-driven" work, and for problem solving.

As one might expect, the development of connectivity has proceeded bottom-up. As of the end of 1992, the international standards for Level 1 are stable and well known. All major hardware vendors have changed their systems to make them connectable to standard networks. The international standards for Level 2 have been defined, but are not widely implemented. Instead, vendors are feverishly working to connect systems through devices that translate from one protocol set to another, and then back again. De facto standards may begin to emerge from these vendor-specific solutions. Routing solutions, even if they do not conform to official OSI standards, are being developed. Much work is being done on Level 3 to define and implement standards for end-user interaction. Although it is getting closer, universal, transparent interoperability is still not available. As stated previously, vendors are developing pragmatic solutions faster than the standards can be defined. Although not all standards have been defined, and many have not been implemented, a completely new industry has arisen lately to provide connectivity solutions at this level. Even though these solutions are not always standards-based,

Table 6.2 Connectivity Questions

Person	Business needs	Connectivity questions
Admitting physician	• Review previous admissions • Review results of pre-admission lab tests • Place orders from a variety of locations • Find location of patient • Access data consistently across all data bases	• Can the physician's Practice Management system be connected to the hospital network? • Can the Practice Management system get across the network to the Lab? To the Pharmacy? To the Medical Records system? • Can the Practice Management system exchange Email messages with the above systems? • Can it extract data from these systems? Can it be updated by these systems?
Pharmacist	• Review previous admissions • Review lab results • Review patient allergies	• Can the RX system access the Reg system? • Can the RX system access the Lab system? • Can the RX system exchange Email with the Practice Management and Nursing systems?
Lab technician	• Review medications • Know changes in patient status (changes in weight or fluid intake)	• Can the Lab system access the Reg system? • Can the Lab system access the RX system? • Can the Lab system exchange Email with the Practice Management and Nursing systems?

they are provided by a new generation of vendors whose business strategy is to connect other vendors.

As stated previously, when the general manager deals with vendors, consultants, and even IS staff, s/he must link standards to business processes and strategy. Once the strategic direction is established, more technical details may be addressed. Many vendors boast that they offer "solutions," but when pressed to match their system to an explicitly defined hospital strategy and architecture, will have difficulty defending their "solution." Table 6.2 frames some of these questions. At the more strategic level, the manager needs to keep in mind long-term goals and critical success factors. (See Table 6.3.)

Potential Counterarguments

Some hospitals might respond that connectivity is not necessary, since their strategy is to acquire all applications from a single monolithic

Table 6.3 Strategic Connectivity Questions

Critical success factor	Activity/ value chain	Managerial questions
Retain profitable admitters	Evaluate physicians	How can the hospital use information technology to assess the profitability and practice patterns of physicians?
	Daily practice	How can information technology be used to make it easier for the physician to practice at the hospital? • Can the physician access hospital information resources remotely? • Can the physician get an integrated view of his patients? • Can we alert the physician when a patient of his is admitted to the hospital?
	Recruit physicians	How can the hospital use information technology to recruit physicians and evaluate their files?
Meet patient service needs on the spot	Registration	How can the hospital use information technology to eliminate mistakes and minimize waiting? • Can all members of the team be connected, so that nothing falls through the cracks? • Can linkages with insurers and employers be set up to accelerate the processing?
	Daily needs	How can information technology be used to meet the complex daily requirements of patients? • Can Nursing find out when some need has not been met by other members of the team, such as Housekeeping or Dietary?
	Discharge	How can the hospital use information technology to eliminate mistakes and minimize waiting?

vendor. Over time, however, this strategy is not feasible, except for perhaps the smallest hospitals. The increasing use of PCs and LANs for specialized applications will continue. This strategy is based on the critical assumption that the hospital's single vendor will design its applications to take full advantage of the single platform (electronic mail, file sharing and access, etc.) many vendors do not. Moreover, the vendor's applications may be too big to fit on a single computer, and so the vendor has to spread them out, and then issues of connectivity arise. Moreover, even if all modules do fit on a single computer, the files might not be integrated. Thus there is no avoiding the need to assess the "connectivity."

A given hospital may have a single vendor, but it will be required to interact electronically through EDI (Electronic Data Interchange) with other entities including vendors, government, payers, physicians, and other hospitals. This is a trend that will only grow.

Even if the hospital employs a single vendor, it still needs to take an architected approach to its business processes and data.

MANAGEMENT DISCUSSION

As with the Business Architecture and the Data Architecture, top management needs to understand the Technical Architecture to a degree of detail that permits effective leadership. Top management, through its involvement with hospital operations, is willing and able to show leadership in issues like TQM and reengineering. With some further preparation, they can pose questions about systems integration and data-driven requirements definition. But mapping network technology to the value chain is an alien discipline to top management.

Top management is generally insulated from the issues of technical architecture, and generally becomes involved unintentionally in ad hoc problem analysis triggered, for example, by a patient's complaint about a billing error, or a doctor's complaint about shared medical record numbers. The CEO may simply delegate all problem resolution to a subordinate. However, most CEOs like to be able to understand the problem to a certain level of detail so that they can explain the situation personally to the complainant. Thus the CEO "drills down" into the specifics, asking "how" and "why" this incident happened. After that, many CEOs will also ask "how" the problem can be fixed. Unfortunately, such questions can lead to technical answers that the CEO does not understand: "Apparently, the Charging system interfaces with the Billing system after midnight, which causes another twenty-four-hour delay in the update of the Collection files. The Lab uses LAT and the Pharmacy uses IPX, so they do not talk."

Top management is unable to pursue this conversation, and simply dictates to "fix it." Unfortunately, many of these "technical" problems are really symptoms of general management problems that go to the core of the organization, and which cannot be resolved by subordinates because they require a redesign that can only be championed by the authority of a CEO. This also happens on a much broader scale, when the CEO is required to make complex, long-term, multimillion-dollar decisions regarding the hospital's use of technology. Not only are the financial stakes high, but the decision affects the strategic position of the hospital, and thus its very survival. Such situations require a comfort level not possessed by most CEOs, and so important decisions are avoided because they are presented in a technical context.

This book does not expect the CEO to micromanage technical decisions. However, if the hospital makes information systems part of its strategy, then it must involve the CIO (VP of IS) in the planning meetings. And the CEO must be prepared to discuss technical issues with the CIO.

Historically, the preferred mode of interaction has been an "arm's length" arrangement: (1) Information Systems is excluded from planning; (2) the CIO functions as a personal translator, with the CEO accepting everything passively; or (3) the CEO relies on a consultant (damaging to morale, does not build internal skills, and allows the CEO to avoid responsibility for IS decisions—the consultant can always be blamed).

In order to provide effective leadership in information systems, the CEO must be comfortable with his understanding of the Technical Architecture. The interesting irony is that the more top management understands, the more effectively they will be able to delegate. The less it understands, the less they will be willing to delegate.

Understanding

Like general management, top management needs a concise, structured way to ask questions and interpret the answers they receive—a "back-pocket" methodology showing how to link strategy to the value chain, how to redesign the value chain, how to discuss the integrating role of data, how to discuss the alignment of technology with business processes, and how to design management controls for all of the above. This methodology can be encapsulated with several of the models discussed previously.

Figure 6.3 reinforces several points: business process interaction and meaningful redesign *within* a business process requires redesign *across* business processes; data is an integrating factor; when one connects the systems *physically*, one needs to determine which business processes need *logical* connectivity. Furthermore, the CEO needs to be able to analyze the control aspects of this new approach to information systems. The Seven S's model summarizes these issues well. It also helps the top manager to assimilate more details, and to structure conversations to maximize understanding of the issues. Thus, the hard decisions on integration will not be put off.

Decisions about information systems no longer lend themselves to traditional cost-benefit analysis. In previous generations of information systems, the benefits were more direct and more quantifiable. Systems were at the operational level and departmentally oriented. They included things like Charge Capture, Billing, Inventory Control, and Payroll. It is relatively straightforward to quantify the benefits of such systems: They allow the hospital to reduce workers; to reduce the consumption of supplies; to do more with the same number of staff, and thus avoid certain expenses; to do more accurate charging. All these benefits can be mapped to the "bottom line" in a simple chain of causality (see Figure 6.7).

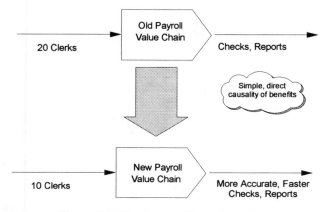

Figure 6.7 Simple causality of benefits.

The new generations of information systems span many departments, if not the whole hospital. To obtain the predicted benefits, many departments need to cooperate. New kinds of activities are receiving IS support, activities whose inputs and outputs are difficult to quantify (market research, managerial decision making). Furthermore, many new applications represent the "infrastructure" upon which other applications will be built. This includes things such as networks, data bases, and productivity tools. The bottom-line benefits of information systems are still quantifiable, but now they are not so direct and immediate. For example, when a hospital decides that one department must change its system to feed an integrated data base, it is declaring that a given department will incur expenses that will benefit another department and the whole enterprise. This greatly extends the benefits causality chain. Or a hospital may decide that all departments must communicate through electronic mail over the backbone network. There will be no net reduction in expenses, but the improvement in service and quality should increase patient and payer satisfaction, which should translate into increased or maintained market share. This further extends the benefits causality chain, since it requires that departments learn to work in concert and that the market will subsequently react favorably to this. Of course, the amount of market share must be assigned a probability, since one cannot be absolutely sure that one's actions will produce the desired reaction on the part of the customer (i.e., increase in market share). The end result is that decisions are made with greater uncertainty, and the impact is more remote, farther downstream in the value chain. In many instances, the benefit decision becomes: "How much is the hospital willing to spend to obtain a particular market share with a particular probability?" In other cases, the decision requires that the hospital take a long-term view of the costs and benefits. This can be difficult, for both financial and cultural

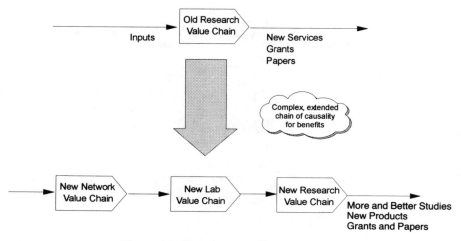

Figure 6.8 Complex causality of benefits.

reasons. Figure 6.8 shows the case where the research activities of the hospital will benefit from the installation of a backbone network, which will allow the extracting of Lab data into a large research data base on the network. Of course, this may require that the Lab collect data in a different way; it also assumes that the researchers will be able to make use of this new, improved data to develop new medical services, which will attract more patients (and bring increased revenue).

Several of these issues are summarized in Table 6.4. Inventory control is a more traditional application, whose benefits are more easily quantifiable and more directly obtainable. A decision support data base is a newer type of system. Its benefits are less direct. It requires that an analyst or manager make a decision, and then that someone else carries it

Table 6.4 Benefit Profiles of Application Types

System	Directness of benefits	Quantifiability of benefits	Potential impact of benefits
Inventory	more	more	lower
	.	.	.
	.	.	.
Decision support data base	.	.	.
	.	.	.
	.	.	.
Backbone network	less	less	higher

out effectively. The backbone network is one of the newest systems, and its benefits are the least direct, since it provides an infrastructure for every other application. On the other hand, the backbone network has the greatest potential to ultimately impact the bottom line of the hospital.

This new methodological orientation of the CEO will permit him or her to request and understand the new kinds of analysis needed to understand the benefits of systems. In earlier times, one could do a cost-benefit analysis at a high level and in a vacuum, without looking at the interaction of the value chains. In accounting applications, such as Payroll, one could simply concentrate on reducing the labor inputs and be fairly confident that the expected benefit of reduced clerical expenses would follow. This is not the case with networking systems.

Leadership

Once a CEO becomes comfortable with the concepts of the Technical Architecture, s/he will be prepared to lead. And, indeed, the CEO will be required to exert leadership, because a structural approach to the business process and information systems requires that the hospital be managed according to new principles. Some of the areas that will require leadership are: setting a vision and building commitment, making hard decisions, dealing with vendors, and managing a new organizational structure.

Vision and Commitment

The idea that systems and processes need to be aligned is still fairly new. And the implications for organizational design are even less appreciated. The CEO needs to have a vision in order to inspire, and an understanding, in order to guide. This vision needs to include information technology.

Difficult Decisions and Trade-Offs

The CEO will have to confront the more complex cost-benefit models of new information systems. Other decisions concern fundamental changes in organizational design and management policies. This can best be achieved through participative management. Sometimes top-down, autocratic decisions are needed to create the momentum for building a new vision and culture, but participative management is needed for its widespread implementation. Participative management means that decisions are not made arbitrarily by top management, hidden from subordinates; it means that subordinates provide frank input and are free to criticize the arguments of top management. Such an approach can be very anxiety provoking for both sides: for subordinates, because they are showing nonconformity, which is not valued in traditional organizations; for top management, because they are abandoning their position of infallibility and admitting that they do not have all the answers. What can greatly help is to have strong models and methodologies. This, once again, shows the value of having a conceptual understanding of the architectures.

Vendor Relations

Top management will have to support technical staff and general managers in their dealings with vendors, who will balk at attempts to measure how closely their systems match the hospital's architectures. A standard such as HL7 allows hospitals to treat the software as components, buying a "core" Registration and Patient Accounting Package from one vendor and then supplementing it with "best-of-breed" niche modules. This presents a threat to vendors, and they will try to discourage this, warning that if the hospital purchases its modules from multiple vendors, then the hospital is responsible for integrating them. Obviously, the hospital has to make a decision that balances functionality against integration. This may require the participation of the CEO. Furthermore, if an integration strategy is adopted, then consultants will be needed. The CEO will have to show leadership in supporting hospital staff in their management of consultants.

Controls

Top management will have to provide leadership in redesigning the organization for the alignment of systems with business processes in a changing competitive environment. This redesign will affect a wide variety of subjects: data policies, systems development policies, funding of system purchases, usage accounting, reward systems, and many more. These topics will be treated more extensively in Chapter 7: Control Architecture.

Data Policies: Conflicts about data ownership and stewardship increasingly require attention, as systems become connected and users gain access to multiple data bases through a single workstation. Individual organizations have stewardship of the data entities, like PHYSICIAN, PATIENT, and CHARGE, which are physically spread throughout multiple systems. But data ownership is something else. PHYSICIAN data such as Name, Doctor Number, and Status of Admitting Privileges belong to the Medical Staff Office, and the authoritative source for this data is the Medical Staff Information System; however, the Physician Name and Number recorded at the time of admission is the responsibility of the Business Office.

Systems Operation Policies: Some departments may desire physical control over their information systems and keep the equipment on their premises. It may turn out that the data in these systems is too critical to the hospital's value chain to leave it in an unprotected environment. Take the example of a clinical information system, whose data base may be used by teachers, researchers, Lab, Pharmacy, and Radiology, as well as for remote consultations. This system should not be in a room without environmental controls such as air conditioning, uninterrupted power supply/battery backup, security, and fire protection. When such territorial conflicts arise, general managers without the proper technical concepts often avoid dealing with these issues.

Systems Development Policies: Some departments may want to do their own systems development. It may turn out that a proposed application is transaction-oriented, high-volume, and affects many departments. In such a case, the hospital must insist that the Information Systems department be involved, to ensure that the proper controls are in place to "harden" the application. In addition, some organization that has knowledge of the strategic plan and architecture must review all large systems projects to ensure that they conform.

Rewards Systems: When systems are managed strategically to provide value across the enterprise, managers must be encouraged to behave for the common good. This means that the hospital's reward system must be changed to reward departments for contribution to common goals. For example, if a project manager suggests doing things that incur budget variances, but which contribute to the architecture, then the reward and measurement system needs to be flexible enough to accommodate this.

Skills and Culture: This organizational redesign also requires new values and skills. Each department must look outside of itself, to see how it impacts other departments within the context of the entire value chain. This requires a non-defensive, non-territorial culture. It also requires that departments be willing to accept some applications that may suboptimize the department, but which are optimal for the hospital as a whole.

TECHNICAL DISCUSSION

The challenge of this section is to present further details of the Technical Architecture without becoming a textbook on the wiring of networks or a side-by-side comparison of individual vendors' products. Both of these topics are worthwhile subjects, and they have been covered elsewhere in more appropriate forums. There are many excellent texts on the topology and wiring of networks; the best vehicle for comparing vendors is the RFP process.

The approach adopted herein is more conceptual. It is directional because it deals with technology trends in general; it does not compare the details of vendor implementations. Vendors are continuously changing their products by upgrading and/or renaming them. Any author who compares systems at a point in time will trigger the protests of offended vendors claiming that the comparison is no longer valid. In light of this, the book develops models that capture the fit between business and technology, and then uses these models as the framework for discussion of the connectivity standards that all vendors need to embed in their products in order to achieve the "fit."

The word "standard" can be used with three different meanings: (1) standards that have been developed and promulgated by official standards-setting organizations such as NIST, ANSI, IEEE, or CCITT; (2) a vendor's convention that has been placed into the public domain as a standard and has been approved by a standards organization; (3) vendor conventions that over time have become a de facto standard, such as IBM's SNA or Novell's Netware; (4) vendor conventions that are not de facto standards. For clarity, "standard" in this book will refer to (1) and (2); "convention" will refer to (3) and (4). An example of a closed system is IBM's SNA. If one wanted to connect to IBM, one had to write their communication software to observe the SNA conventions. In this fashion, many IBM conventions became de facto standards, without IBM ever putting them in the public domain.

This book deals with standards that have a direct bearing on connectivity and integration. It does not treat standards for a wide range of technologies, including (1) hardware (CPU, magnetic disks, CD ROM, printers, bar code readers, etc.); (2) systems software (utilities, programming languages, operating systems, etc.); and (3) applications software (e.g., patient accounting, nurse scheduling, etc.). For example, an optical disk could be used to integrate the operations of the Pharmacy and Lab departments. Its integrating value, however, comes from its use in combination with data base and network software that allows it to be shared.

Conceptual Models

There is a compelling reason for using models when discussing how information systems interact. First, the number of components is very large, and the relationships among them are extremely complex. Next, these connected information systems need to be related back to the business activities that they are supposed to support. Furthermore, the only way to compare systems that have been developed using different models is to use a third model, to which each of the systems can be mapped. Finally, models serve as a "lingua franca," permitting mutual understanding among diverse factions: IS, top management, and end-user departments.

Open Systems Interconnection

In 1977 the International Standards Organization (ISO) and the International Telegraph and Telephone Consultative Committee (CCITT)

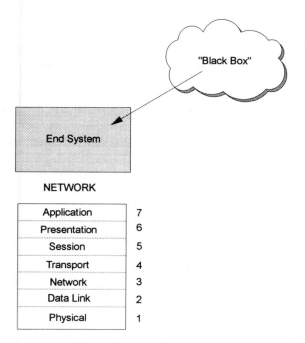

Figure 6.9 OSI reference model.

developed a "reference model" for a "standardized" communications architecture that would facilitate the interoperation of systems using different technologies from different vendors. This architecture is referred to as the "Open Systems Interconnection" or OSI.[1] This model has seven levels or "layers," shown in Figure 6.9.

Each layer of this model deals with a different level of functionality required for an information system to interoperate with other information systems across a network. The design principle is that each end system (or application) is a "black box"; that is, one cannot make any assumptions about how it functions, other than how it interfaces to these seven layers. This allows vendors to maintain their proprietary systems at the application level. The OSI layers are implemented in software, with the exception of layer one. Each layer is insulated from the others by virtue of the fact that it can call only one layer below itself, and can be called only by the layer above it. Each layer can perform one or more related functions, which OSI calls "services." The detailed features of a given function are called "service elements."

---

[1] For a relatively accessible overview of OSI, see Dennis MacKinnon et al., *An Introduction to Open Systems Interconnection*, New York: W.H. Freeman, 1990.

Figure 6.9 is a model for the design of "open systems." That is, if vendors write their application software and system software in conformance with these levels and services, then their systems will be "open"— able to interconnect. In business terms, this will overcome the service discontinuities within the business architecture that are caused by the technology and software design used by the individual applications.

OSI has many different standards groups, working at the various layers of the reference model and in various industries. The committee dedicated to standards for health care systems interoperability is called "MEDIX."

The open systems movement has grown over time, and during 1989–1991 gathered significant momentum, punctuated by the U.S. government's decree that, starting in August 1990, any systems vendor dealing with the federal government must demonstrate that his system conforms to OSI protocols (to the extent that such protocols have been defined). In addition, during 1992 many individual states started to move toward open systems. The European Community too has embraced the principles of open systems. Further evidence is the fact that many vendors are making systems interoperability a business strategy.

Open Software Foundation

It is important to remember that the ISO model was developed at a time when LANs were in their infancy, PCs were unknown, and graphic interfaces were not possible. In addition, there was no concept of portable operating systems such as UNIX. Rather, the pattern was to have large host-based systems with dumb terminals attached. This state of technology greatly shaped the ISO model, which treated end systems as "black boxes," and so it had nothing to say about standards for generic operating systems or user interfaces such as Windows or Motif. It also has nothing to say about the relational model for data bases. Its use of SQL is to pass data from one system to another.

The most significant consortium is the Open Software Foundation, which is attempting to define more explicitly certain components of the architecture of the end systems, which were ignored by ISO.[2]

The complementary nature of OSI and OSF is shown in Figure 6.10. OSF's objective is to augment OSI's goal of "connectivity" with "driveability," portability, accessibility, and manageability. The OSF has analyzed the former black box into four separate areas: management, user interface, system, and data.

---

[2] For a brief, but comprehensive overview of the OSF and its products, see Digital Equipment Corporation, *Open Systems Handbook: A Guide to Building Open Systems*, Maynard, MA: 1991.

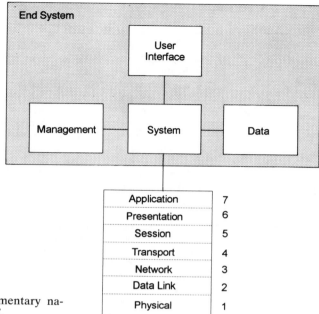

Figure 6.10 Complementary nature of OSI and OSF.

1. *User Interface*: This is the driveability factor: how the user interacts
with the application. This includes ergonomics, forms interaction, menus,
windows, and so on. This relates to the transparency of the application to
the end user.

2. *Management*: This refers to the management of system resources,
including functions such as network security, accounting for use of system
resources, configuration management (what equipment is located where),
and performance management (detection and correction of bottlenecks
and failures). While this aspect is not used by end users, it does directly
impact them, and it is very important to systems professionals.

3. *System*: The operating system, the programming languages, and other
system utilities. This also includes standards for Application Programmer
Interfaces (APIs). Application Programmer Interfaces are standard ways
for programming languages to call operating system functions, user interface functions, or data base functions.

4. *Data*: Data access and interchange. All systems should permit the
same type of data manipulation and transmission. Regardless of how the
data is physically stored, it should be accessed in a standardized way, such
as SQL, and the data resources should be known to all through standardized catalogs. This is different from OSI, which uses SQL only for
data interchange.

Table 6.5 Details of OSI Layers

Layer name	Comment
7 Application	This layer is called the "application" level, but the term can be misleading. Layer 7 provides an interface with end-user applications, but it does *not* provide any actual functionality. At all other levels in the OSI reference model, a lower level provides services (i.e., functionality) to a higher level. For example, if the end-user application is Electronic Mail, then Layer 7 specifies what *data fields* must be passed from one end system to another. It does not specify what the Electronic Mail application does or how it looks to the end user.
	This level provides several "generic" support services: ACSE, ROSE, and CCR. Functional service elements sit on top of these generic service elements (e.g., X.400, X.500, FTAM, etc.)
	The number of functional service elements for Layer 7 is essentially unlimited, since the number of end-user functions requiring connectivity is unlimited. Typical end-user functions that require use of the network are: file transfer, document formatting; data base access; starting a program on another computer; user interface such as Windows; data base integrity; and data base synchronization through standardized transactions.
6 Presentation	This layer performs two major functions: abstract syntax and data representation. "Abstract syntax" is the agreement on which data types will be used, what record types there are, and the sequence of data elements in the records. For example, a protocol may require that a message consist of a record header, a repeating detail record, and a trailer record; and that the header record consist of Sequence Number, Date Stamp, and Sending Institution.
	The second sublayer takes care of translating from one data format into another. For example, IBM machines encode data using the EBCDIC standard, while most other computers use the ASCII standard. It also performs data compression and encryption.
5 Session	This layer, in a sense, is the interface between the network OS the computer's OS. Each dialogue with another machine requires a separate Session. Layer 5 software should allow multiple simultaneous Sessions for a single node. For example, as part of his job, a user may need to be logged onto a clinic scheduling module on host A, while at the same time being connected to a Patient data base on host B. When doing the scheduling, if any questions arise about the patient's address, the user can shift to the Session on host B and change the patient address in the master data base. This layer also performs higher levels of synchronization.
4 Transport	This layer ensures reliable end-to-end communications between Sessions. This layer provides different "classes of service" to the Session. It provides various combinations of functions, including segmenting and assembly of messages, flow control, detection of lost packets, error checking, "connection-oriented" service, or "connectionless" service. It can also

(*Continued*)

Table 6.5 *Continued*

Layer name	Comment
	perform multiplexing. It also inserts the network destination and source address of the message.
3 Network	Layer 3 provides a "best effort" to deliver the data packet, but does not guarantee its correct and accurate delivery (this is the responsibility of Layer 4). The primary function of Layer 3 is to route a message outside of the network to another network, or across an "internetwork."
	It is not feasible to build an enterprise network as a single bus or ring because of distance, traffic loads, and other issues. Instead, they are usually constructed as networks of networks. Therefore, the routing of messages across these intermediate networks becomes a nontrivial task. This layer needs to do the following: (1) determine whether the packet conforms to standards; (2) locate its neighbors on other subnetworks; and (3) determine the best path through the network.
2 Data link	This layer deals with the transfer of a data packet from one node to another on the same subnetwork. (Layer 3 ties the subnetworks together.) Layer 2 specifies how the data will be transferred from a node onto the "data link." The term "data link" refers to the subnetwork. Different network standards have different specifications for how a node is supposed to access the subnetwork and compete for its resources.
	In a "bus" network, every node is located along a logically linear cable, called a "bus"; a message can be broadcast by any node at any time, and all nodes are listening. The message travels along the cable until it is sensed by the appropriate node; all the nodes are listening in, and the target node senses its address and takes the message. In a "ring" network, every node is located on a logical ring. The order in which nodes transmit is controlled by a logical "token."
	There are two major sublayers: LLC and MAC. The LLC (Logical Link Control) is medium independent and performs error detection and recovery. The MAC (Medium Access Control) specifies the electronic signaling characteristics of the subnetwork. In a sense, it is the interface between the LLC and the Physical Layer.
	Many of the terms at this layer are commonly associated with Layer 1. Many people use "802.3," "X.25," and "FDDI" to refer to both the signaling characteristics of the network and the physical characteristics of the cable.
1 Physical	Specifies the different types of physical cabling media that will be used by the Data Link protocols. This could include coaxial cable for Ethernet (802.3), Token-Ring (802.4) or Token-Bus (802.5); twisted pair (telephone wire) for Ethernet, Token-Ring or Token-Bus; RS-232E cable for X.25; or fiber for any of the above. Standards will soon be published for wireless networks (which use radio waves or infrared waves as the transmission medium).

The *network* is the traditional connectivity services of the OSI reference model. The four "end system" components are connected to the network by a series of APIs—the way that these different programs call the network resources.

Recently, there has been a movement by vendors to form standards "consortiums." This has been spurred by the growth of interest in standards, the "commoditization" of hardware, advances in LANs, PCs, GUIs, and operating systems. As part of this, the vendors are offering their own products and conventions as the standards to be implemented. The potential advantage of this is that standards can be developed sooner, and in a way that is geared toward implementation. The danger is that this process will unfairly bias the standard in a vendor's favor. The other danger is that the vendors, driven by their own interests, will not be able to agree and will disband, having wasted resources and distracted the attention of the standards-setting bodies. This has already occurred with the Distributed Computing Environment (DCE), which consisted of DEC, Compaq, and other well-known vendors.

Details of OSI Layers

Table 6.5 presents the details of the OSI's seven layers.

Recall that in the general discussion a network was divided into only *three* major layers: network connection, network routing, and end-user functionality. This was a simplification for expository purposes, but a valid one. Layers 1 and 2 deal with access to the immediate subnetwork. Layers 3 and 4 deal with routing and end-to-end management of the message. Layers 5, 6, and 7 deal with the operating system and the end-user application that needs to interoperate.

Any given layer can only communicate with the layer immediately above and the layer immediately below. In addition, there are rules for how these calls may be performed. This layering insulates a given layer from changes that are made in another layer. For example, one may work on enhancing the functionality of electronic mail while one introduces new algorithms for routing messages across networks; all this while installing a new physical cabling system. This neat division into calling and called layers is nothing new. Good software design has always done this. However, there was never a common design according to which vendors could develop their software. Historically, vendors have developed their own proprietary software, with their own proprietary functional design, so that any given level of vendor software is liable to combine several OSI layers, or vice versa. At the same time, the vendor features bear little resemblance to the service elements defined by OSI.

The standards have been defined and implemented "bottom up." For example, the standards for physically connecting a system to a network (Layer 1) have been developed before standards for data base access

(Layer 7). This is not surprising, since it is fruitless to talk about file exchange if there is no common network mechanism for transmission of the data.

While the OSI model is conceptually simple and elegant, there are many practical problems. OSI terminology is extremely abstract, and that abstractness creates confusion for the lay reader who is not steeped in the methods of object modeling and abstract syntax notation. In addition, some layers are so complex that they must be divided into sublayers. Not all of the eventual functionality has been specified. Finally, OSI standards are just high-level logical specifications for programs, not the programs themselves. Much depends on how vendors implement these specs. If vendors implement the specifications incorrectly or inconsistently, then the objectives of the OSI model will be frustrated.

Finally, there is the question of "packaging" these standards. OSI standards are not monolithic. At any given layer, there is a choice of standards. A given company or industry will use only a subset of the OSI standards, which are quite numerous. There needs to be a way to combine multiple levels of standards into a "package." This is in the process of realization, and is called ISP (International Standards Profiles). These profiles combine the standards for electronic mail, file transfer, session management, routing, and physical connection for a given industry.

Functional Scenarios

Any discussion of the OSI model must include concrete examples to compensate for its abstract terminology. Assume a Pathologist working in a large hospital that has a heterogeneous computing environment. He is one of many people who need transparent access to multiple data assets (others include medical researchers, auditors, strategic planners, and a variety of clinical practitioners). As this Pathologist is reading the test results of a patient with a nonspecific diagnosis, he recalls that he has seen similar patterns among other patients. He requests that the Lab System retrieve all patients with this diagnosis and these test results for the past two years. After he gets this, he decides that he would like to know more about their family histories and cases, so he retrieves the history and physical (H&P). He also accesses the Pharmacy system to obtain detailed data on the medicines they were taking. He thinks he has come upon a valuable insight, and so he writes a memo to a colleague in a neighboring hospital in the same medical center, and he attaches a copy of the X-ray and a spreadsheet with the statistical calculations. He mails this memo and moves on to another research topic. Table 6.6 summarizes the connectivity standards needed to support this complex activity.

Figure 6.11 illustrates the Email portion of this scenario. The pathologist's Email application calls an API that produces a standards-based message (using X.400 and X.500 for global naming). Layer 6 takes care of

Table 6.6 Connectivity Standards Needed by Business Activity

View lab results and incorporate into an Email document

Activity	Standard
Work with multiple computers	• Session protocol • Data conversion • Routing • Network connection • RPC to run program on another computer
Access the patient data base and extract those patients that meet the selection criteria	• SQL for data extract • Distributed Data Catalog
Review many forms of data	• Protocol for user interface
Send a memo and attach a complex report and statistical analysis to the memo	• Complex document architecture standard • Email (types of fields, features like "cc:") • Logical "global" naming for addressing anyone on any network

encryption (if this is an issue). Layer 5 associates the message with a network session. Layer 4 maintains the end-to-end integrity of the message (packaging, stopping and restarting). Layer 3 maps the logical name of the recipient to the physical address of the adjacent router. Layer 2 prepares the physical frame of bits that will be sent. At Layer 1 the stream of bits is sent onto the network. The routers on the internetwork route the message using tables. If the protocols of the end systems are different from the intermediate network, they are either translated or encapsulated. The receiving system (the other researcher) executes the same steps, in reverse order.

OSI Stack

Publications on OSI frequently refer to the "stack." A "stack" is a list of program instructions that may be processed top-to-bottom (LIFO) or bottom-to-top (FIFO). The significance of this metaphor for OSI is that its functional levels are implemented as software and are executed either top-to-bottom (transmitting systems) or bottom-to-top (receiving systems).

The easiest way to understand the OSI stack is to examine how a minicomputer provides connectivity services to its attached terminals. When the end-user application needs to communicate with other end-user applications, it notifies the minicomputer's operating system, and the operating system calls other software modules that control sessions, data formatting, routing, and so forth. This is illustrated in Figure 6.12, which shows the activity of the Registration Clerk. When a patient is readied for admission, the clerk, who is logged onto the Registration system, checks to see whether the patient has been admitted to the hospital previously,

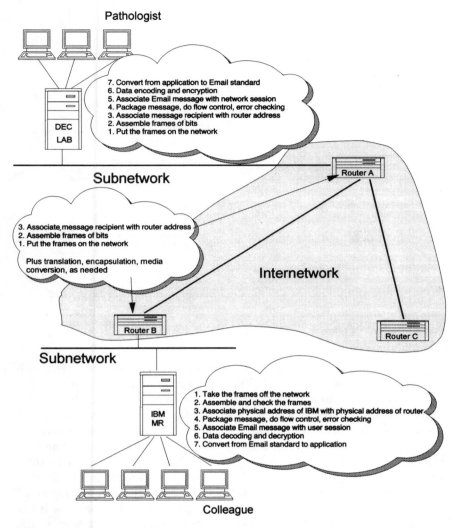

Figure 6.11 Pathologist-Colleague interaction at OSI layers.

assigns a Medical Record Number, verifies insurance, enters the admitting diagnosis, assigns a bed, and stores the record in the data base on the local minicomputer. As the admission record is being stored, the Registration system broadcasts this admission to all interested systems (e.g., Lab, Pharmacy, etc.). It does this by requesting network access from the operating system, and the operating system calls a series of subroutines (the stack) to format the message correctly and manage network communication.

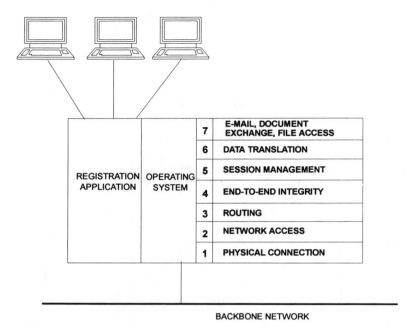

Figure 6.12 Registration clerk and the "stack."

The stack can thus be represented as a program structure chart, with "calling" and "called" modules. This has been done in Figure 6.13. Each box represents a module of functionality—a service. Higher level functions call lower level functions. The interface between any two levels consists of a program call and a parameter list. Those modules above the heavy line represent the end-user application; those below the line represent modules in the network stack, which have been keyed to their respective layers in the OSI model. For example, "format transaction" is marked with "7," indicating that it deals with a Layer 7 service. Table 6.7 provides more commentary on this. The interface into the network is the module "Store in Remote Data base." Each layer accepts data from the higher (calling) layer, adds its own data, and passes this expanded data packet downward. The end-user data comes from the application. All the other data that gets added is protocol-related (OSI calls them "PDUs"—protocol data units).

This type of analysis is valuable for any network, regardless of its OSI status. These layers of functionality could be implemented through non-OSI protocols. Good software design requires that developers modularize their system's functionality into layers.

In reality, the stack is probably spread over several components of the minicomputer. In a workgroup LAN connected to a backbone network, the software modules of the stack are distributed over multiple components. Figure 6.14 shows a PC attached to a LAN, whose LAN server

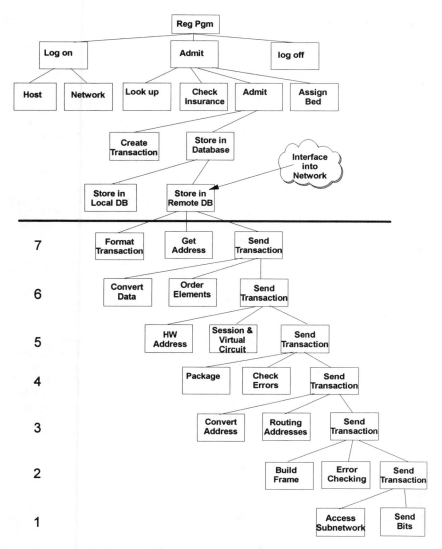

Figure 6.13 The "stack" as a program structure chart.

has two network boards. One connects to the LAN; the other serves as the gateway to the backbone network.

OSI versus Vendor Protocols

Historically, each major hardware vendor developed its own proprietary networking system. This was understandable, for both technical and

Table 6.7 Commentary on the Stack's Layers

Subroutine	Layer	Comment
Registration		
Log on	n/a	The user logs on to his host computer for the day,
Admit		and spends most of his time admitting patients.
Log off		At the end of the day, he logs off. His host is
		attached to a backbone network that employs a
		connectionless scheme, like Ethernet. Part of
		the admitting activity consists of broadcasting
		the admit data to other systems that have
		patient demographic data.
Admit		
Lookup	n/a	The major functions within Admitting are:
Check insurance		checking to see whether the person has been
Admit		admitted to the hospital before, checking for
Assign bed		valid insurance, the admission itself, and the
		assignment of a bed.
Store in DB		
Store in local DB	n/a	When a patient is admitted, the admission
Store in remote		transaction is first stored on the application's
DB		host CPU. Then it must be sent to all other
		systems that require admissions data.
Store in Remote	7^+	
DB		
Format trans		*Format trans*: The HIS vendor maps his data
Get address	7	elements and segments into the data elements
Send trans		and segments that are required for the HL7
		transaction. Layer 7 of the stack accepts these
		elements. Note: Layer 7 does not provide any
		services; rather, it simply accepts the fields
		from the end-user application.
		Get address: The stack has a global naming
		functionality. Layer 7 maps the names
		supplied by the HIS vendor to a logical name in
		the global directory.
		Send trans: Request the services of Layer 6.
Send Trans	7	
Convert data		*Convert data*: Layer 6 converts the HL7 data
Order elements	6	from one encoding scheme to another; for
Send trans		example, from EBCDIC to ASCII.
		Order elements: It also provides a syntax notation
		that indicates the end of a segment, optional
		elements, repeating groups, etc.
		Send trans: Request the services of layer 5.
Send Trans	6	
H/W address		*H/W address*: Assign the port number of the user
Session	5	originating the message.
Send trans		*Session*: Layer 5 associates the message with the
		appropriate session, adding this information to
		the packet. The Admitting Clerk might have
		several different network sessions
		simultaneously—one for broadcasting updates,
		and another for Email messages.
		Send trans: Request the services of layer 4.

(*Continued*)

Table 6.7 *Continued*

Subroutine	Layer	Comment
Send Trans	5	
Package		The system now calls a series of routines that
Check errors	4	eventually result in the physical transmission of
Send trans		the HL7 message. The Transport Layer (4) performs end-to-end packaging functions. It separates the higher levels from the details of the physical subnetworks over which the message travels. The Network Layer (3) provides routing information. And the Data Link Layer (2) builds the packets and sends them out over the physical network.
		Package: Segment the HL7 transaction at one end, and then reassemble it at the other end. The HL7 message might be broken down into multiple sub-messages. These are not necessarily the same size as the physical packets that eventually get transmitted at Layer 2.
		Check errors: The Transport layer provides error checking, like "checksum," to provide end-to-end message integrity. Older systems had less reliable transmission media, and so did more error checking at layers 2 and 3. As the physical network becomes more reliable, the error checking can be done at layer 4.
		Send trans: Request the services of layer 3.
Send Trans	4	
Convert addr		*Convert addr*: Add physical network address of
Routing	3	the host.
addresses		*Routing Address*: Builds in routing information,
Send trans		by associating the message with the "next hop" in the physical subnetwork. It takes the global logical name and determines the physical addresses and best route.
		Send trans: Request the services of layer 2.
Send Trans	3	
Build frame		*Build frame*: Break the data down into smaller
Error checking	2	packets (frames) of data that can be
Send trans		accommodated by the physical characteristics of the network. For example, a single HL7 transaction might be too long to be contained in a single packet.
		Error Checking: Compute a check sum and include it in the frame.
		Send Trans: Layer 2 sends one of the frames of the HL7 transaction.
Send Trans	2	
Access		*Access Subnetwork*: The physical medium is
subnetwork	1	acquired for access.
Send bits		*Send Bits*: The electrical pulses move onto the cable.

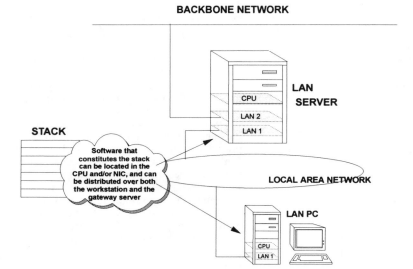

Figure 6.14 Distribution of the "stack."

business reasons. During the 1960s and 1970s there were no independent standards for networking. This technical vacuum had to be filled by proprietary products from the vendors. Besides filling out the vendor's product line, the products bestowed another advantage: They tended to lock customers in to the given vendor. Incompatibility of hardware and software creates a major obstacle to acquiring products from other vendors. This incompatibility, which arose by chance, was then consciously perpetuated. Vendors became unwilling to release the specifications of their products, or to make them compatible with equipment from other vendors. While all vendors faced this conflict between their self-interest and the interest of the customer, IBM raised this to an art form. (IBM has since abandoned this practice.)

Over time, the situation has changed. Vendors have been forced to move toward standards, largely because of the growth of TCP/IP, LANs and the "commoditization" of PC hardware. LANs demand connectivity and interoperability. As their margin for hardware shrinks, vendors are beginning to add higher-margin products such as software, services, and special connectivity hardware such as routers. They are also adding standards-based software to their product lines. Vendors are moving from being exclusionary to accommodating heterogeneous networking.

Table 6.8 compares selected OSI protocols with vendor conventions and de facto standards. IBM and DEC are prominent among vendors whose proprietary conventions served as de facto standards: IBM, because of its dominance in the computer industry until the mid 1980s;

DEC, because of the strategic direction it took with distributed computing in the early 1980s. However, the Internet has produced the most common de facto standard with its TCP/IP. This book deals with three "standards" for backbones: Systems Network Architecture (from IBM), DEC Network Architecture (from DEC), and TCP/IP.

The word "standard" is frequently used to signify one of three different approaches: official standards promulgated by standards-setting groups; de facto standards (vendor conventions that have been adopted by many vendors); and "standardizing" devices, which could be either hardware or software that translates from one standard to another. For example, X.400 and X.500 are ISO standards for electronic mail. A de facto standard is Novell's MHS convention. A "standardizing" device would be a software bridge that translates from DECmail to PROFS. At a lower level, there is routing.

Table 6.8 shows how difficult it can be to try to compare functionality across vendors. A given vendor's convention will rarely match the OSI standard one-to-one in features. The naming of the services does not help determine comparability. In addition, the services encompassed by the vendor's product are likely to span several OSI layers. (This lack of feature isomorphism and layer mixing prevents the easy mixing and matching of protocols—they are definitely not "plug and play" yet). For example, the functionality provided by the NetBios protocol (and program) spans Layers 4 through 7 of the OSI stack. The same is true of the NFS protocol from Sun Microsystems. TCP/IP, while it literally refers to Layers 4 and 3 respectively, also encompasses protocols at Layers 5 through 7. While SNA has seven levels, their content and purpose differ significantly from the seven layers of OSI. The different protocols have different capabilities. DECnet allows the routing of messages anywhere across a network of networks. TCP/IP also has this capability. NetBios does not. SNA has static routing. TCP/IP has dynamic routing. All this further reinforces the need to have a reference model such as OSI.

Table 6.8 refers to several protocols not previously discussed. They concern data base access, Document Exchange, File Concurrency and Recovery, and Remote Procedure Calls. They represent additional aspects of interoperability. Remote Data base Access has specifications beyond those of File Exchange, including record level access. Document Exchange builds on Email standards, but also includes specifications for how to embed graphics within the document. Remote Procedure Calls allow the originator of the message to explicitly call a program on another computer.

Figure 6.15 presents these issues in three concrete systems. How can a hospital structure these systems so that they behave according to the logic of the business? The Registration process is supported by a system running under IBM's SNA. The Laboratory is supported by a system running under Digitals' DECnet. The Pharmacy operation has a system that runs

Table 6.8 Comparison of Protocols

OSI layer	OSI service	OSI protocol	IBM	DEC	TCP/IP and other
Application	User interface	POSIX	SAA/CUA	NAS/ DECwindows	Windows (MS)
	Electronic mail	X.400, X.500	PROFS	All-in-One	CEO (DG) SMTP (TCP) MHS (Novell) NFS (Sun) FTP
	Remote data base access and file transfer	FTAM	RDA, SQL	DAP, DFS	
	Document exchange	ODA/ODIF	DCA	CDA	
	Industry-specific transaction exchange	MEDIX, MAP/TOP, X.12			HL7, MMS Vendor-specific interfaces
	File concurrency and recovery	CCR			NFS
	System management	CMIP	Netview	DECmcc	SNMP (TCP) Open View (HP) AFP (Apple) Named Pipes
	Remote procedure calls	ROSE	APPC/LU6.2		
Presentation	Data encoding syntax	ASN.1	SNA	DNA	NetBios
Session	Management of the dialogue between two end systems	ISO 8327	SNA	DNA	NetBios

Layer	Description		SNA	DNA	
Transport	Data integrity of the message, packaging the message for transmission	CONS (Connection-oriented Services CNLS (connectionless services)	SNA	DNA	XNS (3COM) TCP IPX/SPX (Novell) NetBios Appletalk
Network	Routing of message packets across subnets	ISO IS-IS ISO ES-IS X.25	SNA	DNA/LAT	XNS IP IPX/SPX/RIP (Novell)
Data link	Access to the immediate subnet, transmission from node to node	X.25 HDLC 802.2 802.3 802.4 802.5	Bisync SDLC	DDCMP	Arcnet Starlan Asynch
Physical	Electrical and physical characteristics of the immediate network	FDDI EIA-423 RG-59 coax RG-62 coax	Twinax (AS400)	Twisted pair/ MMJ	Twisted pair Coax

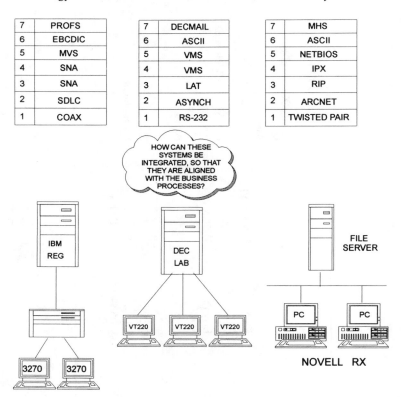

7	PROFS
6	EBCDIC
5	MVS
4	SNA
3	SNA
2	SDLC
1	COAX

7	DECMAIL
6	ASCII
5	VMS
4	VMS
3	LAT
2	ASYNCH
1	RS-232

7	MHS
6	ASCII
5	NETBIOS
4	IPX
3	RIP
2	ARCNET
1	TWISTED PAIR

Figure 6.15 Three nonintegrated systems.

under Novell's operating system. It can be seen that, at each level, the components of the supporting systems are incompatible, making it impossible to support the integrative activities of the hospital.

1. *Electromechanical Component*: The plugs and wires are different, so they cannot be physically connected to the same cable. IBM uses RG-59 coaxial cable; the Novell system uses twisted pair (telephone wire); and the DEC system uses RS-232 (a cable containing 25 wires).

2. *Network Component*: Each system accesses its network differently. IBM's SNA uses a protocol called SDLC for data transmission: a simultaneous two-way exchange of data, brokered by the host computer. DEC's Asynch is one-way-at-a-time exchange, brokered by the host; Novell's Arcnet is one-way-at-a-time, but requires an acknowledgment; there is no host that brokers the transmissions from user stations—it is token bus. IBM's SNA is oriented toward hierarchical communications. DEC and Novell are oriented toward peer-to-peer.

3. *Message Component*: Each system has a different format for the sending of messages. This includes the addresses of the sender and receiver, as well as features like "priority," "acknowledgment," and "cc:".

4. *Routing Component*: The packet sizes and error-checking methods are different. So is the addressing and routing of messages. There is no common scheme for setting up and managing a session on another host.

5. *Data Component*: IBM encodes its data as EBCDIC; DEC and the PC use ASCII.

6. *File Component*: At the application level, there is no common way to access the data on another host. DEC uses RMS to access and manipulate its files; IBM uses VSAM (Virtual Storage Access Method); and Novell uses B-trieve. (Actually, RMS, B-trieve, and VSAM are not part of the OSI stack. They are on the application side and use services embedded in the overall network operating systems.)

7. *Other Components*: They differ for all aspects of interoperability: file transfer, message exchange, document exchange, and system management.

Systems Network Architecture

This is IBM's standard for enterprise networking. Work on SNA started in 1974, long before the advent of personal computers and LANs. The initial goal of SNA was to link IBM mainframes and their terminals. It has since been broadened to connect IBM's "strategic" platforms: 3090 mainframes, AS/400, RS/6000, and PS/2. Superficially, SNA resembles the seven layers of OSI (see Figure 6.16); however, they differ sub-

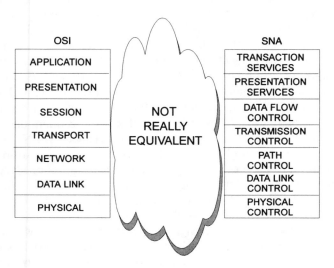

Figure 6.16 Superficial similarity of OSI and SNA.

stantially. SNA is not really an open architecture; it expects, even demands, to be connected to only IBM devices (homogeneous network). OSI assumes multiple heterogeneous vendors, and so its layers have more complex and numerous features at all levels, particularly at Layers 3 and 4. At Layers 3 and 4 IBM's Path Control assumes that only IBM systems form the intermediate network between two end systems. At Layers 1 and 2 IBM assumes the existence of a "connection": fixed packets with determined arrival times, and acknowledgments. Other networks such as OSI allow for "connectionless" transmission of data. Historically, IBM desired to guarantee levels of service with this deterministic type of network. IBM was hierarchical; other vendors were peer-to-peer. There was no provision for routers and bridges among multi-vendor networks.

For a long time, IBM actively discouraged the use of Ethernet, Novell LANs, UNIX, and other de facto standards. The growth of TCP/IP, inexpensive, powerful PCs, and local area networks have eroded IBM's ability to dictate the use of SNA. And so, around 1990, IBM began to open up SNA, allowing direct Ethernet connections, collaborating with Novell, and making SNA more amenable to peer-to-peer networking (critical when one's display devices are no longer dumb terminals but PCs). IBM is now in the process of changing its front-end processors so that they can attach to bus and ring backbone networks as peers, rather than as upward concentrators.

Over the years, third-party vendors have "opened up" SNA by creating gateways to it. These gateways have allowed asynchronous terminals to access SNA networks, other computers to run programs on SNA hosts, and users to exchange electronic mail with SNA users.

OSI has incorporated individual IBM protocols (such as RDA and SQL). SNA was originally a hierarchical network, reflecting the architecture of host, front-end processor, and terminal. All traffic had to be moved upward, to the FEPs, before it could be transmitted horizontally. In the late 1980s IBM began to moderate its strategy of closed hierarchical networking. For example, IBM has made TCP/IP and Ethernet controllers available internally for its machines. Moreover, it is developing devices that will offload more network functions from its hosts and their front ends, changing its APPC/LU6.2 protocol to accommodate a wider variety of network nodes. This new protocol is called APPN (Advanced Peer-to-Peer Networking) and it will accommodate peer-to-peer networking and multi-protocol routing, including translation of SNA instead of tunneling. It will be interesting to see how quickly IBM can shed its hierarchical mentality. IBM is also changing other Level 7 conventions, such as SAA. SAA (Systems Application Architecture) is a set of standards and tools for software design and development that was supposed to allow the software to look the same and run on all of IBM's strategic hardware platforms. It appears that IBM is moving away from its own conventions toward established standards for user and programmer interface, such as X-Windows.

DEC Network Architecture

Originally, DEC's networking was closed. In the last several years, however, DEC has modified DNA so that it will converge with the OSI model. DEC's clustered approach to distributed processing, as well as its historical requirement to connect with IBM, have contributed to this positioning. DEC has promised that Phase V of DNA will merge with OSI. Actually, DEC has redesigned its network operating system to support three parallel stacks, DNA, OSI, and TCP/IP (see Figure 6.17). This appears to be a reasonable migration strategy; however, management of network nodes that are at different stages of conversion could be a problem. A backbone network supplied by DEC could provide the gateways to other vendors that are at various stages of migrating to open systems. These gateways could include SNA and TCP/IP. However, the reader should not assume that DEC has reached the stage of "plug-and-play." This will not occur before 1997.

DEC has had a tradition of nondeterministic networking, like Ethernet, but has moved to provide native support for deterministic networks such as Token Ring. IBM, which historically used deterministic networking such as SDLC has lately moved to support nondeterministic networking like Ethernet. Rather than trying to provide the "ultimate" NOS, DEC is positioning its network software as the glue that will hold together a wide array of NOS's, allowing them to interoperate.

TCP/IP

TCP/IP is a vendor-independent protocol, originally developed by the Department of Defense to connect governmental agencies involved

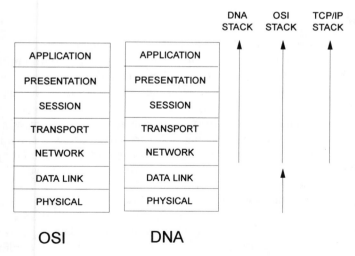

Figure 6.17 OSI and DECnet.

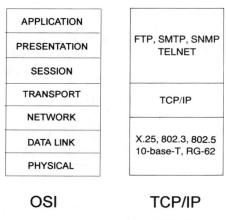

OSI   TCP/IP

Figure 6.18 OSI versus TCP/IP.

with national defense. It is heavily used by educational institutions and aerospace manufacturing as well.

Strictly speaking, "TCP/IP" stands for "Transmission Control Protocol/ Internet Protocol." TCP and IP are two different protocols, at Layers 4 and 3, respectively. TCP is a Transport Layer protocol that ensures reliable delivery of messages (datagrams). IP is a Network Layer protocol that allows TCP message segments to be routed among different networks. In addition, TCP/IP also includes a suite of protocols that correspond to the higher layers of the OSI model. They include: FTP (file transfer), SMTP (electronic mail), Telnet (virtual terminal protocol), and SNMP (for network management). See Figure 6.18

MUMPS

MUMPS deserves special discussion. Developed in the late 1960s, MUMPS was originally totally monolithic—it was a programming language that also performed the functions of a data base management system, an operating system, and a network operating system. This monolithic approach to systems architecture runs contrary to current trends, which separate application software from system software, and which further separate networking software from systems software. In that era, however, there was no other way to build a distributed system. Data base management systems and networking systems were in their infancy; there were few software tools.

With MUMPS, the hospital bought a "closed" system, and was dependent on a single vendor for all functionality, both application and connectivity. In recent years the MUMPS programming language has been separated from its operating system features. Some MUMPS applications can now run under other operating systems using standard network protocols. In many cases, however, the MUMPS data base management system has been retained. In order to make this open, it must be given an SQL front end. There are many dialects of MUMPS. If a hospital is thinking about acquiring a MUMPS application, it should make sure that the application is written in the MUMPS language, but it does not need the complete MUMPS environment to run.

Others

Historically, network operating systems came from the major hardware vendors. Their original focus was to give a terminal user access to multiple host computers—all from the same vendor. In the 1980s other vendors of network operating systems began to emerge. These operating systems were much easier to use, even though they had limited functionality. They were PC-oriented, and their developers were not major hardware vendors. They included companies such as Microsoft, Novell, Banyan, and 3COM, and a host of third-tier companies. Some used a client-server model; others did "peer-to-peer" networking. Their original purpose was to connect PCs in a Local Area Network, providing file services, print services and electronic mail. They were all proprietary at first.

Over time, Novell has become the de facto standard. Their design was for work groups and departments, not for total enterprises, and so their Layer 3 and Layer 7 protocols were weak or nonexistent. Their session support was weak. They could support only a limited number of users. They did not possess global naming. This has started to change, so that the following pattern is emerging: Traditional mainframe and mini vendors are approaching OSI functionality by adding PC services and greater internetworking; PC vendors are approaching OSI functionality by adding global naming features, greater number of users, and internetworking.

At the same time, there is increasing activity among third-party vendors who supply layer 1 through 3 products for internetworking and network segmentation: hubs, bridges, routers, multi-protocol routers, and so on. A second group of vendors wants to ensure Layer 7 functionality across multiple platforms and insulate the application from all the network details. For example, a vendor of a distributed relational DBMS has software that will run on a variety of CPUs. However, in order for a user to access this distributed data, the user must be able to get across the internetwork and then call the DBMS program on these remote computers. The problem is that not all these vendors have the software to allow this, so the DBMS vendor provides a standard API, which then calls "middleware," which provides the Layer 4 through 7 functionality.

The above represents an overall trend to "componentize" the network, illustrated in Figure 6.19. For example, Novell provides the LANs; DEC provides VAX clusters; UNIX machines are used for data base servers;

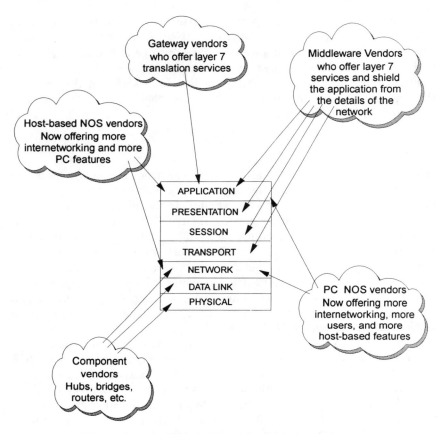

Figure 6.19 Multiple levels of network development.

still other vendors provide the internetworking devices that hold it all together.

Connectivity Solutions

The Appendix to this book provides a survey of different connectivity architectures that have arisen at different points in time. The architectures are examined using the three applications of Registration/Patient Accounting, Laboratory, and Pharmacy. Recall the different types of hospital users of information systems: managers, data-driven analysts, "heads-down" users, and clinical users (physicians and nurses). The technology is evoluated for its ability to support their needs. The OSI model is used as a point of reference.

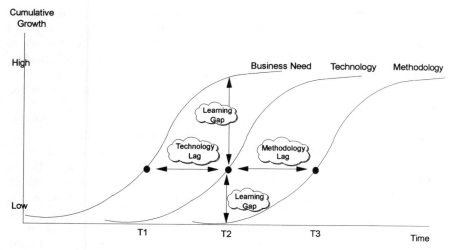

Figure 6.20 Learning curves and technology adoption.

The evolution of these architectures shows the constant interplay of business need, technology, and methodology, discussed in Chapter 3. New business requirements emerge from a changing environment and the competitive initiatives of industry rivals. Business needs exhibit a growth curve similar to that of the learning curve. In Figure 6.20, for the curve labeled "business need" the vertical axis represents the cumulative number of companies that have perceived a business need. Initially, a few companies realize how the balance has changed, and they move to adapt to the changed environment. Over time, more and more companies react to the change. Eventually, most companies adapt. Obviously, the late adapters now occupy a weak competitive position. (Some hospital chains did not appreciate how much the industry was changing in the early 1980s, and they continued their acquisition policies right up through the introduction of DRGs in 1983. Their competitive position was negatively affected by their lag in learning.)

The same pattern can be seen in Figure 6.20 for technology adoption. The vertical axis represents the cumulative number of companies adopting a technology for a business need. Some companies sooner than others realize that a given technology can be useful. The earliest adopters are not necessarily in the best competitive position, since the early phases of a technology can be expensive and unreliable. Generally, a hospital should adopt as soon as possible, depending on its position in the industry as a whole and vis-à-vis its particular segment rivals. (In some instances, there are valid reasons for not adopting the technology: The hospital has compensating strengths; rivals do not intend to use it; the hospital has no capital; the segment simply does not require it; not all changes in the business environment require a new technology.) Nevertheless, a "lag" occurs between identification of the business need and introduction of the technology. The longer this lag, the higher the opportunity costs for the hospital. In "high tech" medicine, the business need *is* the technology.

A similar curve can be observed for methodology. The term "methodology" refers to the effective use and management of technology. It is not enough for the hospital to introduce a given technology; it has to develop methods for its use and management. Once again, a gap occurs between the spread of the technology throughout the hospital and the growth of methods for its use and management. These gaps are illustrated in the architecture examples in the appendix.

The challenge is to shorten these lags and reduce the oportunity costs. Otherwise, a hospital will be in the position of trying to understand technology 1 when it is on the decline, while it should be concentrating on technology 2. The examples in the appendix deal with some technologies that are old but that continue to be used (and even adopted). Similarly, having the newer technology is no guarantee that a hospital has a methodology for its effective use.

Physical Networks

While a backbone network, such as in Figure A.8 (Appendix) is intended to create the impression of logical unitry and transparency, it itself does not have to be monolithic, in either media or protocols. When a network is designed, it is usually divided into segments and subnetworks, as shown in Figure 6.21. (However, in most cases the hosts would be consolidated in a data center.) Segmentation is done for several reasons: performance, ease of management, and security. Fault isolation, wiring, and expansion are easier to do when there is segmentation. In many of the constituent LANs 90 percent of the traffic may be local. Security on heterogeneous networks is difficult to implement and manage.

A network segment might be a floor, a whole building, a particular work group. It is a defined region, bounded by routers, which keep some traffic off the "backbone." For example, a departmental network generates much traffic that is destined only for a member of that particular department. The department might generate large graphics files that need to be transmitted to another building. Rather than put this onto the backbone, the hospital can route it onto a special fiber segment. A backbone can consist of multiple media: coaxial cable, twisted pair, fiber cable, and wireless transmission schemes such as microwave and radio frequency.

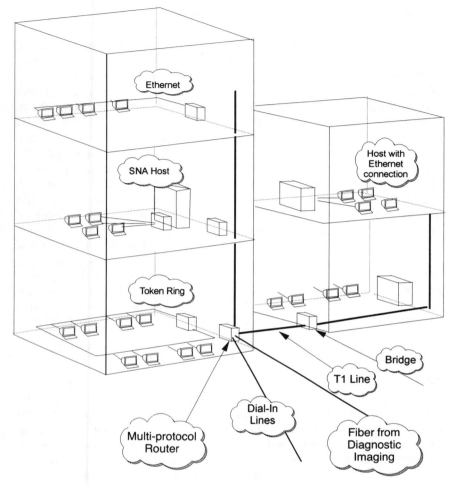

Figure 6.21 Network segmentation.

When organizations tie their LANs together across cities, they do not achieve the speed and reliability of a local backbone. The existing standard of X.25 is proving inadequate for the throughput required by modern backbones. This, however is changing quickly. Third-party carriers are moving to link LANs over digital lines using protocols such as ATM and ISDN. ATM in particular will address the requirement that a backbone should be able to accommodate the aggregate traffic generated by the segments and subnetworks. For example, if three 10-Mbit LANs are connected to a 10-Mbit backbone, the potential aggregate demand is 30 Megabits.

Evolving Solutions and Architectures

The 1990s are seeing intense activity in product development at all seven network layers. Previous generations of systems dealt mostly with traditional "data processing" data—the structured text and numbers of record-based files. Now other data modalities are being integrated: images, video, sound, and unstructured text. This greatly improves the fit between systems and business processes. Integration over an area wider than a campus is becoming possible with improvements in WANs. Traditionally, lack of connectivity, reliability, and throughput have been obstacles to integrating WANs. New transmission media and protocols eliminate these obstacles. The trends to simplify organizations, to link organizations, and to tighten service and control cycles all demand this increased throughput and ease of connection. There is also increased demand for tools to manage all of this from a central location. Installation and management are becoming simpler. The overall trends: Layers 1 and 2 are seeing greater speed and reliability through new media; Layer 3 is seeing greater routing capability; Layers 4 through 6 are being made less intrusive for the users; and Layer 7 functionality is greatly expanding. In five years, Layers 1 through 6 will be taken for granted by everybody.

Layers 1 and 2

At Layers 1 and 2, new transmission media and protocols are being developed. This includes wireless transmission using radio waves or infrared waves, fiber optics, and improved techniques for transmission over copper wire (digital networks such as ISDN and ATM). Other protocols include Frame Relay and SMDS (Switched Multimegabit Data Services). As these technologies are developed, they will require gateways to existing Layer 1 and 2 products. Management of these diverse technologies is becoming easier as vendors develop devices that allow all these media and protocols to exist within the same piece of equipment. Multiple segments and types of LANs, together with WANs, will all coexist in the same box ("backbone in a box"—see Figure 6.22).

Another satisfying aspect of all this new technology development is that it is being done in a more standards-conscious way. Individual vendors are submitting their technologies to standards bodies for official adoption as standards; or consortiums of vendors working on a technology are submitting it as a de facto standard supported by multiple vendors. The approval process is slow—there are not enough standards-testing organizations—and the consortiums can be undermined by vendor interests and the inherent flaws of consortiums. Nevertheless, the overall process is producing integrative products at a faster rate than ever before.

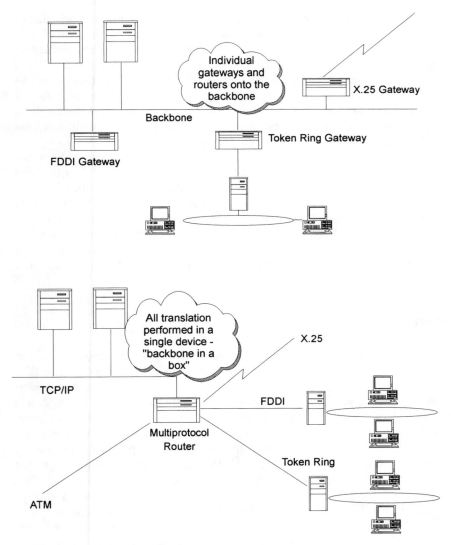

Figure 6.22 Backbones and routers.

Layers 3–7

Advances will be made in routing over multiple subnetworks. These developments pave the way for innovative restructuring of business processes within and across companies. Multi-protocol routers will give way to "multidimensional" gateways: devices that will translate virtually from anything to anything at all network layers. These devices will have a global name server which will have a detailed profile for each name, listing the network the person is on and his/her software profile. The gateway will thus know whether it has to translate from one protocol to another. For example, if a user desires to send a Novell-formatted Email message to some other user, the gateway will know whether it has to translate the protocol. Eventually, the world will get to more fundamental OSI implementations of networks, whereby devices use OSI standards as their "native" protocol. In the meantime, however, vendors will continue to build more powerful translating devices.

Over time, as standards become more universal and management becomes easier, there will be less need to focus on the physical details of the network, and data issues will come to the fore. Layers 1–6 are necessary for integration of business processes, but not sufficient. Data, whose services and standards are at Layer 7, is the key to logical integration. In the early 1990s, despite the advances in object orientation and heterogeneous data bases, too little attention is paid to the data aspects of companies—logical data models, data distribution, data ownership, and so forth.

OSI Networks

The architectures discussed in the Appendix are analyzed within the framework of the OSI model, but they use few OSI protocols. The OSI model specifies conceptually the network services and the levels at which they should be provided. Interoperability in Figures A.6, A.7, and A.8 is achieved through gateways. A gateway is simply a device that performs protocol translation at one or more levels of the stack. This is in contrast to a "bridge," which merely converts from one physical medium to another; or a "router," which selects the best route for the message, but which does not necessarily translate from one protocol to another. The trend, however, is to offer all these features in a single device. Gateways are at Layer 3 and above. Actually, they can be divided into three types: Layer 3 (Novell to SNA); Layer 7 (from PROFS to All-in-One); or layers 4–6 (e.g., session management). This last type is often referred to as "middleware." Gateways can be stand-alone (dedicated to a single type of translation) or combined. For example, vendors of heterogeneous DBMS's (designed to provide access to multiple vendors' data bases distributed over multiple hardware platforms) frequently bundle all the different types of APIs into their DBMS, to shield the customer from the details of the network.

Gateways have both advantages and disadvantages. The advantages are: (1) The hospital can achieve connectivity faster, using multiple de facto standards, rather than wait for fuller implementation of OSI by vendors; (2) the hospital's existing investment is preserved by the acquisition of relatively inexpensive hardware. The disadvantages are: (1) translation consumes a lot of resources and can degrade network performance (Ethernet, for example, assumes that a message will travel from one end of the network to the other in a fixed number of microseconds); (2) queuing and processing in gateways can add delays longer than the signal propagation time; if the same computer is used for both end-user applications and gateways, the application will slow down; (3) there is no guarantee of insulation from the changes made to vendor products, and there is no independent testing body; (4) like human language translation, something is frequently lost in the process—features and functions on one side of the gateway may not have analogs on the other side.

Parallel Protocol Stacks

If the whole world could suddenly shift to OSI standards then there could be a single protocol stack. This will not happen any time soon, so a viable vendor strategy is to have *multiple* stacks, rather than do third-party translation. This would push much of the processing back onto the host computer or PC network interface card, but it might speed up the process by eliminating gateway queues. This is illustrated in Figure 6.23. The top half of the diagram illustrates the strategy of translation. When the Pharmacy user wants to access data on the Lab's machine, the Data General Computer builds its own network packets and sends them to the gateway, which either converts them to backbone packets or wraps backbone protocols around them ("tunneling"). At the other end, the process is reversed.

The bottom half of Figure 6.23 presents a dual protocol stack. When the Pharmacy user wants to query data in the Lab system, the user changes sessions; the second session is associated with the OSI stack. Instead of translating or encapsulating, the host computer itself directly builds an OSI packet. The OSI stack could be thought of as another Novell NLM. Some vendors (DEC, NCR) have made such dual protocol stacks part of their strategy. The disadvantage is that dual stacks also consume resources (but so do gateways, and gateway queues are more harmful to network performance). Extra memory is required to store and run them. Translating is most convenient for vendors in the short run, because they do not have to redesign their operating systems.

Vendor Steps to Open Up Systems

While the trend to adoption of standards started in the late 1980s, most HIS products on the market were developed years before that. Vendors have difficulty opening up their systems because they were never designed with a modular separation into levels of network functionality, or, if they

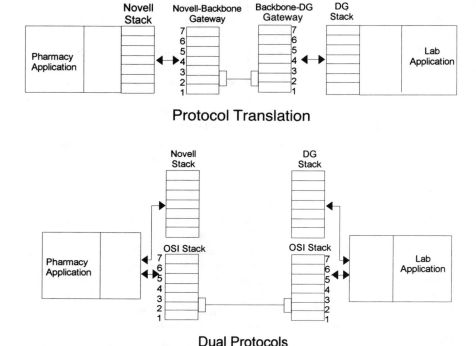

Figure 6.23 Protocol translation versus dual protocols.

were, each vendor used their own type and number of levels. This results in the following problems: (1) The vendor may not have the ISO specified function; (2) the given function may be performed at the wrong level; (3) the function may not have the same set of features as that specified by ISO. For example, a vendor may have file transfer capabilities, but places them at a different layer, or does not provide the same file attributes as those specified by OSI.

Hardware Vendor

The CPU vendor traditionally supplied both the host operating system and the network operating system. In many cases there was no clear separation of the two. Now, the CPU vendor must modularize the system's functionality according to a layered scheme. This means restructuring the operating systems to allow the user to maintain multiple network sessions using multiple protocols. The operating system must provide an API for a windowed user environment. Other APIs include Email, remote procedure call, file transfer, and so forth. This entails rewriting the routines that call the network functions, including a "standard" stack in addition to the vendor's proprietary stack. In the case of a LAN that is gatewayed onto the backbone, one stack would be used for communications within the LAN; the other would be used to exit onto the backbone.

This situation presents the CPU vendors with a terrible dilemma: The more software standards they implement, the more their hardware becomes a commodity. The ultimate in user flexibility would be to run a portable operating system, such as UNIX, which could be moved, along with its applications, from one vendor's machine to another's. The vendors see this and are developing new value-added products, which include gateways, integration services, and network management software. DEC is moving into software and integration services, DG is becoming the low-price seller; IBM is trying to use APPN as a way to use its SNA networks as backbones.

Utility Vendors

The concept of "utilities" is broader than the traditional utility programs like Sort and Merge. It includes those activites that are common across a wide range of application programs (electronic mail, data base access, remote procedure calls, and system management) and which require interaction among systems. They will have to be rewritten to conform to standard APIs. Electronic mail must accommodate the X.400 and X.500 protocols. Tools for monitoring the network's equipment and throughput must be able to exchange data according to the standards of either SNMP or the OSI CMIP.

DBMS Vendors

Data Base Management Systems must be changed to conform to the Client-Server model. For vendors of traditional host-based DBMS's, this means moving some functions down to the PC and workstation (or other host). Vendors of PC-based systems will have to move all the data management functions up to the server. This means rewriting most of the APIs. Implicit in the Client-Server model is the requirement that the DBMS hand off the records to the NOS for delivery across the network. This means removing any network functions that have been designed into the software. In reality, Layers 4–7 have not yet been standardized and/or implemented on a wide basis, so vendors whose DBMS's run across multiple platforms are forced to bundle these layers as "middleware" with their DBMS software. While doing this, they need to provide a dual-stack capability, so that they can run on open networks.

The DBMS needs to provide an SQL front end, which accepts remote queries using RDA. The CCR (Currency Control and Recovery) protocol, which provides for two-phase commits when data base updates are made across a network, is not necessarily desirable in a hospital environment. A two-phase commit requires that all systems update their data base; otherwise they all will "roll back" the transaction. In a life-and-death situation, with a critically ill patient, it is not prudent to insist that all systems be updated at the same time. Some vendors have an alternative method for data base commits that accommodates such situations. DBMS's must also support a distributed data catalog, whereby each physical system has a complete copy of the logical schema of the data base and a pointer to where the data is physically stored.

HIS Software Vendors

Application software should not perform functions below Layer 7. This would include session management, address management, or packetizing of messages. They also should not perform the generic Layer 7 functions such as Email, data base calls, and so on. Some HIS vendors may still have network addresses "hard-coded" into their application. In other cases, the application vendor may directly manipulate some obscure features of the hardware, without going through the operating system. Many vendors have their own proprietary standards for data base synchronization, not HL7. Some vendors write their applications to run on terminals with special features. Many also write their own file back-up routines. These features can be quite powerful and useful, but, they should not interfere with connectivity, and the vendor should provide the hospital with the option of turning off that feature and using another, less powerful one, for the sake of connectivity. This is similar to the concept of a dual protocol stack.

More and more hospitals desire to have a standard "health care workstation" whereby all applications have a similar look and feel. This issue is not so important for "heads-down" users, who perform the same function every day, or for institutions with a monolithic vendor. However, this is very valuable for users who must spend large amounts of time with multiple applications that run on multiple platforms. In order to do this, most vendors will have to rewrite their screen input and output routines to conform to a standard API.

As vendors redesign their products to conform to standards, they continue to protest that such standards stifle innovation. This claim is an oversimplification. Rather, the standards "channel" innovation and enhance connectivity, which can suffer from innovation. The constant flow of new technology is not always worth adopting, and it distracts hospitals from their "methodology lag" (see Figure 6.20) Hospitals currently have more technology available than they can assimilate. Most hospitals would benefit if they de-emphasized technology development for a year and focused on standards development and reengineering of their business processes.

Application vendors face the same dilemma as hardware vendors: the more standards they employ, the more they are like commodities, allowing a hospital to purchase a single module, rather than the whole system. However, this gives them the opportunity to enrich their programs with application-specific functionality, rather than waste resources on common connectivity features.

Hospital Steps to Open Up Systems

The reader should recall the reason for opening up information systems—to make them more adaptive so that they can be aligned more closely with the Business Architecture, which can change frequently. If a hospital adopts a strategy of aligning systems with processes, it can adopt one of three approaches: (1) It could discard its existing systems and start OSI de novo; (2) it could retrofit its existing systems; or (3) it could place gateways among its existing systems. There are many valid reasons for a hospital not to commit to OSI initially: (1) a desire to retain its existing systems investment; (2) risk aversion, given the evolving state of the standards; (3) it can't wait for functionality in OSI products, it needs the functionality now; (4) OSI is too theoretical, not pragmatic enough; (5) the hospital staff do not have the requisite skill sets.

The most reasonable approach is a gradual migration combining features of each of the following: (1) Demand open features for new applications and systems; (2) work with vendors to modify existing applications; (3) use de facto standards like SNA or TCP/IP instead of OSI; (4) use gateways and other conversion/coexistence products; (5) plan for the replacement of "legacy systems."

Legacy systems are the hospital's oldest information systems, which typically have been written in an older technology with few or no open features. Much of the data required by other systems is captured by legacy systems (which is why they were developed first!). There is little that can be done to retrofit them. But some connectivity features can be "superimposed" on them. For data base synchronization, if a legacy system can output its transactions in any format whatsoever, they can be sent to a third-party server which will convert them to HL7 format and send them to the other interested systems, and to a decision support data base as well. One could also use MS Windows to capture the transaction from the screen and send it to the server.

Implementation of "Open" Systems

After it has adopted its systems strategy, the hospital needs a methodology for implementation, with the following steps:

1. Link strategy, value chain, and connectivity features

2. Develop architecture and standards

3. Develop a migration plan

4. Issue RFPs

5. Implement projects

The business strategies must be mapped to the value chains that impact their success. And the value chains must be mapped to connectivity features; this reveals which "open" features are most important to the hospital. These open features will be ensured by defining a systems architecture and standards. Using this architecture, together with the existing configuration and prioritized business projects, the hospital develops a systems migration plan, implemented through a series of projects. (A warning: the hospital must be prepared to change this plan if major changes occur in technology or in the business environment.)

1. Link Strategy with Value Chain

A hospital might determine that long-term trends dictate that it adopt the strategies outlined in Table 6.9. It would then map each strategy to one or more Critical Success Factors—the things that must go right in order for the strategy to succeed. These critical success factors are realized by one or more business processes, whose interactions must be supported (i.e., they have connectivity needs). Table 6.10 shows the results of this analysis. Eventually, the value chain of each business process will be examined.

The hospital staff that perform these high-impact processes have connectivity requirements, shown in broad outline in Table 6.11. For each

Table 6.9 Hospital Strategies

Strategy	Critical success factor
Mega medical center	• Attract the best clinical talent • Achieve the best cost/quality/ satisfaction • Get patients in and out easily
Total quality	• Record data quickly and accurately • Maintain close-knit teams • Retain qualified staff
Managed care	• Know the costs of each service • Predict patient utilization • Measure resource utilization
Prevention	• Develop and maintain new channels • Obtain community cooperation

Table 6.10 Connectivity Needs of Business Processes

Strategy/critical success factor	Business process	Connectivity
Mega Medical Center		
• Attract the best clinical talent	• Research • Clinical activities	• All patient data accessible from single workstation • All data accessible to physician office
• Achieve the best cost/ quality/satisfaction	• Interdepartmental team problem solving • Documentation of activity • Case review	• Email
• Get patients in and out easily	• Registration • Discharge planning	• All patient data accessible from single workstation • Email
Total Quality		
• Record data quickly and accurately	• Order entry • Medication • Vital signs • Charting	• Synchronization of all order data • All patient data accessible from single workstation
• Maintain close-knit teams	• Interdepartmental team activity • Scheduling	• Email
• Retain qualified staff	• Staff training	• All data accessible to physician office
Managed Care		
• Know the costs of each service • Predict patient utilization	• Track labor costs • Track inventory • Track patient encounters	• Access to all cost data • Access to all patient encounters, across all departments and longitudinally
• Measure resource utilization	• Track orders • Track procedures	
Prevention		
• Maintain new channels	• Home treatment • Treat in office • Treat in clinic	• All sites on the same network • Email
• Obtain community cooperation		

user, one needs to build a detailed map showing the required data and whether s/he is the creator or user of that data. (See Table 6.12.) In most instances, the data will be duplicated across multiple systems, which will require synchronization transactions. Table 6.13 contains a matrix for analyzing the advisability and feasibility of automated synchronization.

Table 6.11 Connectivity Map of Users

User	Location	Activity	Transactions/connections	Frequency, volume, system availability
Lab technician	Main Bldg Room M204	Results analysis	Connection to Pharmacy system and HIS	25/day 24 hrs/day Short transactions
Physician	Medical Office Bldg Room 220	Admitting	Access to HIS when making changes to data base	5/day 10 hours/day Short transactions
Admitting clerk	Main Bldg Room 103	Admitting and Scheduling	Connection to Scheduling system	50/day 10 hrs/day Long transactions
Clinical researcher	Medical School Room 218	Analysis of disease trends, treatments, demographic trends	Connection to all clinical and administrative systems, as well as external data bases	10/day 10 hrs/day Very long transactions
Biller	Admin Bldg Room 110	Send claims to payers	Email with payers Connection between Patient Accounting system and EDI system	50/day 10 hrs/day Short transactions
Pharmacist	Main Bldg Room 130	Check for allergies and interactions	Connection between Pharmacy system and Lab system	35/day 24 hrs/day Short transactions
Outpatient clinician	Outpatient Bldg 220	Clinical activity	Connection to Registration, Lab and Pharmacy systems	30/day 10 hrs/day Short transactions
Radiologist	Main Bldg Room 125	Reading of X-rays	Connection to Lab and Pharmacy systems	50/day 24 hrs/day Short transactions
Strategic planner	Admin Bldg Room 310	Analysis of patterns in costs, practice patterns, demographics, physican statistics	Email Connection to all systems	5/day 10 hrs/day Very long transactions

Table 6.12 Users and Creators of Data

Creator \ User	Registration	Billing	Med recs	Laboratory	Pharmacy	Radiology	ICU	ER	Nursing
Registration		ADT data Demo data	ADT data Demo data	ADT data Demo data	ADT data Demo data	ADT data Demo data	ADT data Demo data	ADT data Demo data	ADT data Demo data
Billing	Bill data Payment data								
Med recs	MD data	Charge		MD data	MD data	MD data	MD data	MD data	
Laboratory		Charge	Results		Results	Results	Results	Results	Results
Pharmacy		Charge	Medication	Medication		Medication	Medication	Medication	Medication
Radiology		Charge	Reading	Reading	Reading		Reading	Reading	Reading
ICU		Charge	Procedure						
ER		Charge	Procedure						
Nursing				Nurse Notes	Nurse Notes	Nurse Notes	Nurse Notes	Nurse Notes	

Table 6.13 Feasibility Matrix for Connectivity

Synchronization	Frequency and volume	Criticality of synchronization	Ease and cost of automating	Controllability of manual process
Med Staff system → Reg system • Physician updates	1 add/month 3 chg/month 30 adds in Sept	• Alienation of MDs • Lawsuits • HCFA problems • JCAHO problems	• $40K for PC side	Fairly easy
Reg System → Lab System • Patient Demographics	30 IP/day 100 OP/day	• Admission delays • Treatment delays • HCFA problems • JCAHO problems	• $40K for REG • $20K for LAB	Quite difficult, particularly for OP
Pt Accting → Radiology • Charge items	1 add/month 1 chg/month	• Payer problems • HCFA problems	• $40K for Pt Accting • $20K for Radiology	Fairly easy

Not all data base synchronization must be automated immediately, or at all. For example, there may be a Medical Staff data base running on a local area network, which has the authoritative data for all hospital physicians. Many other systems have physician data (in particular, Name, Specialty, Admitting Privileges, and Physician Number), and receive manual notification of changes, adds and deletes. The data may be sufficiently low-volume, sufficiently static, or difficult to integrate. One of the problems with existing LAN technology is that it is built on top of DOS, which does not really provide multi-tasking and fault tolerance. If one is sending real-time updates to multiple data bases, one needs these features.

This matrix analysis could be continued, mapping users to data, data to systems, and so on. Obviously, this cannot be done without automated tools.

2. Develop Architecture and Standards

The network must have blueprints and standards. The standards specify what may be used at each level of the 7-layer model. The standards are reinforced by policies and procedures, which ensure that departments conform. There is occasionally a need to issue a "variance" from the architecture for certain critical applications, but the policy would specify that a plan be devised for the eventual conformance of this "deviant" application. These issues are discussed at length in Chapter 7: Control Architecture.

A large portion of the architecture comes from the data architecture and the business architecture. The results of the data collection and analysis are contained in Tables 6.9–6.13. Against this context, the hospital develops the details of the technical architecture. This means selecting topology and medium. What protocol should be used: Ethernet, Token Ring, Arcnet, FDDI? This depends on the nature of the traffic. Will the traffic consist of short, "bursty" transactions; will it consist of frequent large file transfers; does the time of arrival of the message need to be guaranteed; will images and/or graphics files be transmitted? Do you want to combine multiple data types over the same wire? Should the network be wired as a linear bus; should it be hub and spoke? What is the impact on reliability and management? Will portions of the network be segmented for performance and security reasons? What about the medium: coaxial cable, twisted pair, microwave, fiber?

Determine how individual subnetworks will access the backbone and be routed over it. This involves the use of bridges, routers, and gateways. Establish standards for internetwork routing and data integrity (Layers 3 and 4). They may be SNA, TCP/IP, or OSI protocols. Install gateways between the backbone and other networks. Segment the network for performance, installing bridges and routers where needed. There may be some departments that have heavy intradepartmental data exchange. There is no need for them to send all their transactions over the backbone. Extra wiring and routers can be used to check addresses so that only extra-departmental address transactions go from the subnet to the backbone.

Determine whether existing applications will run over the backbone. There is no guarantee that an application designed to run in a host and terminal environment will run over an Ethernet across a gateway: for example, can a user with a PC access the HIS from a LAN, while the application was originally designed to be run over vendor-specific cabling with a dumb terminal? The hospital must be wary when a vendor claims that his product runs over "Ethernet." This may only hold true for Layer 1—the electromechanical properties of the cabling systems—while the vendor may use proprietary protocols for Layers 2 and 3, which would prevent other systems from interoperating with it. Systems may *physically* share the same cable, but have no *logical* interaction.

With regard to Data Architecture, the hospital must develop a catalog of the data and its keys; tools for data management; a design for the physical placement of data bases; policies on their ownership, interfaces, and how the enterprise data gets synchronized; and prioritization of which systems need an automated update and which systems can get along with a manual update.

3. Develop a Migration Plan

Every hospital has a portfolio of "legacy systems" that do not conform to the architecture. There will have to be a short-term plan for accommodating them, and a long-term plan for replacing them. The hospital has two levels of migration efforts—the infrastructure level (Layers 1–7) and the application level (the "black boxes" above Layer 7).

At the network level: do you replace the departmental applications with the backbone; do you keep the departmental networks; if so, how should they be gatewayed onto the backbone; do they even need to be gatewayed onto the backbone? At the application level there are several issues: transactions, data base, user interface. For transactions, how can the hospital keep the data base updated and synchronized with all the other hospital data bases? If a data base is not easily accessible, create a strategy for cloning it into a larger decision support data base. With regard to user interface, how will users be given a single "window" into the information resources of the hospital? How can applications and nodes do Email, document exchange, and other connectivity functions? There are also security and management issues to consider.

4. Issue RFPs

The hospital will need to make all Requests For Proposals "enterprise aware" by including connectivity questions based on the 7-layer model (see Table 6.14). Both hardware and software vendors, sensing that momentum is building for open systems, will respond that their systems are open, so the hospital needs to ask *how* this openness is implemented. A useful technique is to specify connectivity scenarios based on the data in Tables 6.9–6.13, asking the vendors how their systems would support each scenario. The application vendors will protest that they have no control over the network; conversely, the network vendors will protest that they have no control over the applications. In this fashion they can whipsaw the hospital that does not have extensive in-house skills. One approach is to use the services of a systems integrator, who will guarantee that the individual components connect with each other as specified in the RFP. However, over time, more and more vendors are willing to act as the integrator.

Standards for Health Care Data Exchange

If the network is the physical glue, then the data model is the logical glue that holds everything together. The data model requires that multiple data bases be synchronized. This is done through electronic data interchange. Standards for electronic data interchange have been growing in all industries. EDI permits just-in-time inventory control, electronic payments, shared product specs, and a variety of other interorganizational linkages. The traditional "interfaces" of HIS vendors are an example of *intra*organizational EDI. There are several standards for health care data exchange. Some of them are competing; some are complementary. They are:

- *HL7* for the exchange of ADT data, charge data, and orders and results.
- *MEDIX (IEEE P1157)*: for all hospital data.
- *ASTM E31.1*: for lab data reporting.
- *ACR-NEMA*: for the exchange of imaging and radiology information.
- *MIB (Medical Information Bus—IEEE P1073)* for the exchange of the physiological data generated by monitoring devices.

HL7 and MEDIX both deal with traditional structured HIS data: admissions, charges, orders, discharges, and so on. MEDIX is the official OSI effort, international in outlook. HL7 is rather an ad hoc vendor-dominated effort, mostly limited to the United States. In terms of scope of data, HL7 is a subset of MEDIX. The two organizations have created a group that is working to achieve convergence of the two efforts. Eventually, HL7 will be subsumed into MEDIX. Several of these standards are discussed in detail below.

Health Level 7

In March 1987 the HL7 Working Group was established. This committee, which consists of both users and vendors, is trying to standardize the format and protocol for exchange of key sets of data between/among health care applications. The HL7 spec has gone through a series of releases as it is broadened and refined. The most recent is 2.1. The issues are:

- Definition of data to be exchanged;
- Timing of interchange;
- Communication of errors to the respective applications.

The HL7 standard addresses interfaces among systems that might send or receive ADT data, orders, results, and billing data. This standard could eliminate the need for complex custom interfaces among systems. With data exchange standards, if the hospital has N systems, then at most it has to maintain N+1 interfaces; however, without such standards, it might have to support as many as N(N-1) interfaces. With standards, the

Table 6.14 RFP Questions by OSI Layer

Layer	Functionality	Standard	Questions
Above 7	Integration	n/a	Will the application vendor handle all integration?
	User interface	POSIX	Application vendor: Will the application work under Windows on a PC?
			Network Vendor: Will the network run as a Windows task?
	Network management	CMIP, SNMP	What protocols are used for management of the application's network?
			Can this network be controlled from the backbone network? If the protocols are different, is there a gateway?
7	Remote data base access	ANSI SQL	Does the application use a DBMS? Is this a third-party DBMS?
			Does this DBMS have an SQL front end that supports remote access by applications on other networks? If so, what Session and Transport protocols are supported? What interprocess communications protocol is supported?
	Electronic data exchange	MEDIX/HL7	Does the application provide a standard set of HL7 transactions? If so, are they batch or real-time?
			Does the application require a particular type of network, or is it neutral with regard to the network selected? What type of interprocess communication is required?
	Electronic mail	X.400/X.500	How does the vendor provide X.400 Electronic Mail services? If not, does s/he have an X.400/X.500 gateway? Is this a two-way gateway?
			Does the network support global naming? Can the user customize this global name?
	Remote job execution	ROSE	Can a user of this network start another job on a different network?
	Terminal emulation	Telnet	Does the application require the use of a special terminal? It should be able to send data streams for display on a variety of standard devices.
6	Syntax	ASN.1	Does the application exchange data with ASN.1 notation?

(Continued)

Table 6.14 *Continued*

Layer	Functionality	Standard	Questions
	Encryption	DES	Does the application allow data encryption before transmission over the internetwork? If so, what encryption protocols are used?
5	Management of dialogues among end systems	Telnet	How many network sessions may an individual user have? Is this number limited by the terminal, by the application? Does the vendor support? How does the HIS application behave when the end user is trying to maintain multiple dialogues with multiple systems? Does the vendor allow both connection-oriented and connectionless services? May the user have simultaneous sessions on different types of networks? What "middleware" is available?
4	End-to-end data integrity, flow control	TCP	How does the network handle the end-to-end guarantee that messages have integrity and are synchronized? What "middleware" is available?
3	Routing over intermediate systems	IP	Can the application's network be connected to other types of networks? Can a user who resides on a different network access this application? How? Does he need a second network connection, or may he use a gateway? Are the gateways two-way? Can a single gateway support multiple protocol conversions?
2	Access to immediate network	802.3, 803.5	Does the application run over different network protocols? If so, how many network protocols are supported? Are they standard? (Some vendors use the term "Ethernet," while in reality they use Ethernet cabling at Layer 1 and a proprietary protocol for Layer 2)
1	Hardware characteristics of immediate network	10-Base-T FDDI	Does the application require a particular type of cabling (it should not)? May the hospital "bridge" the network from one physical site to another? Does the vendor provide bridges from one physical medium to the other?

Table 6.15 HL7 Trigger Events for ADT

• Admit a patient	• Update patient info	• Pending transfer
• Transfer	• Patient departing	• Pending discharge
• Discharge	• Patient arriving	• Swap patient
• Register O/P	• Cancel admit	• Merge patient information
• Pre-admit	• Cancel transfer	• Response by query
• Transfer I/P—O/P	• Cancel discharge	
• Transfer O/P—I/P	• Pending admit	

addition of a new system requires one new interface; without standards; it could result in as many as N new interfaces.

The HL7 model consists of the following: (1) trigger events, (2) messages, (3) segments, and (4) data elements. The messages and their associated segments are specified as "transaction sets." There are different types of trigger events specified for each functional area. Table 6.15 presents the trigger events for ADT.

The occurrence of an event—a patient admission—will "trigger" a synchronization message, which is sent to all the systems that have a "stake" in that data. A "stakeholding" system is one that also contains the entity—or entities—in question. A message containing patient demographic data is thus sent from the ADT system to the Laboratory, Pharmacy, Billing, Radiology, and so forth. Obviously, one application "owns" the data, while the others use it. ADT owns it, since it is the first system to capture it. The message contains several segments: a Patient ID segment and a Patient Demographic segment. The message also contains segments with control data. Each segment has data elements.

The following represents an Admission event:

"Patient William O. Jones, III was admitted July 18, 1988 at 11:23 A.M. by doctor Sidney J. Lebauer (physician # 004777) for surgery. He has been assigned to room 2012, bed 01 on nursing unit 2000."[3]

This event, marked by the addition of a new record in the Registration data base, triggers a message that is sent from the Registration system at the MCM site to the Lab system, also at the MCM site. The message could be sent in real time, or held until the end of the day. In this case, it is sent on the same day as the admission, but with a three-minute delay. The transaction to be passed consists of the Message Header

---

[3] Example adapted from a working paper containing a preliminary draft of HL7 version 2.1, HL-7 Working Group, *Health Industry Level 7 Interface Standards*, version 2.1, 1990.

Message Header Segment

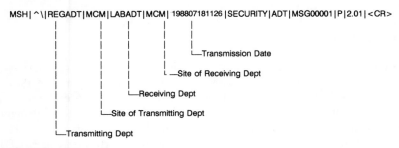

Event Type Segment

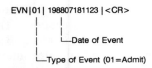

Patient ID Segment

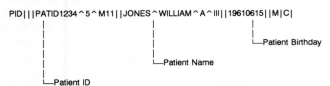

Figure 6.24 Structure of HL7 transaction.

Segment, the Event Type Segment, and a Patient ID Segment, shown in Figure 6.24. The messages for Charges and Orders would have a similar structure.

HL7 does not require any particular type of physical network. It can run over an Ethernet, Token Ring, or an asynchronous connection. It does not have to be real time; it could be run in batch. Unlike MEDIX, however, HL7 does not intend to propose a "suite" of protocols for interoperability, spanning all seven layers of the OSI model. HL7 also differs from MEDIX in that MEDIX has a global model for the inter-operation of systems, and MEDIX is an officially sanctioned committee of the Institute of Electronic and Electrical Engineers (IEEE). HL7 is very oriented toward implementation. Moreover, it is somewhat vendor-dominated, and one can get the impression that the committee is throwing "everything but the kitchen sink" into the standard, so that vendors will not have to change their systems. However, its weaknesses are its strengths. MEDIX has been in existence for the same period of time, and has been slower to define and implement any standards. The plan is for MEDIX to use HL7 as a prototype and to eventually subsume HL7. The two organizations have set up a "convergence subcommittee," to ensure that they do not diverge.

MEDIX/OSI

This committee was started by a group of health care systems professionals gathered at the Medinfo conference in 1986. It was sanctioned in 1987 by the IEEE as P1157, the Committee on Medical Data Interchange.[4] Its goal is to define standards for the interoperability of heterogeneous health care information systems. Its scope is thus broader than that of HL7, which is concerned with the narrower issue of interfaces. The MEDIX committee is more academic in its background and its approach. They rely heavily on object-oriented modeling and abstract syntax notation. They are developing both a transaction model and a data model. The transaction model is based on state diagrams and object modeling. The HL7 committee, on the other hand, is more practical and implementation oriented. MEDIX is also less vendor-influenced.

Rather than reinventing the wheel, MEDIX uses existing OSI protocols insofar as they exist. It is trying to assemble these standards into an ISP (International Standards Profile). An ISP is a suite of protocols, spanning all seven OSI layers, used together to provide connectivity for a given functional area or industry. An ISP thus provides a total connectivity solution. In the manufacturing industry MAP (Manufacturing Automation Protocol) and TOP (Technical Office Protocol) are examples of ISPs. The health care industry needs a "HAP" (Health care Automation Protocol). A hypothetical HAP, shown in Table 6.16, might include: MEDIX transactions, X.400/X.500 for electronic mail, FTAM for file transfer, RPC for executing remote jobs, SQL for data access, ISO Session and Presentation protocols, ISO connection-oriented protocol for the Transport layer, ISO IS-IS and ES-IS for the Network layer, and 802.3 for the Data Link layer. Because Layers 3–7 are still evolving, a more practical HAP can be found in Table 6.17. It relies on proprietary middleware to insulate the application from the network. It uses the de facto standards of SNMP for management, TCP/IP for routing, and Windows for user interface.

Transaction Servers

Some vendors provide a node that receives all the synchronization transactions, and then distributes them to the interested nodes. This is the

---

[4] For an overview, see John J. Harrington et al., "IEEE P1157 Medical Data Interchange (MEDIX) Committee Overview and States Report", *Proceedings of the Fourteenth Annual Symposium on Computer Applications in Medical Care* (IEEE Computer Society Press, 1990) pp. 230–234.

Table 6.16 Hypothetical Health Care Automation Protocol

7	MEDIX, X.400, FTAM, ROSE, SQL
6	ISO Presentation
5	ISO Session
4	ISO CONS, CNLS
3	ISO ES-IS, ISO IS-IS
2	802.3, 802.5
1	10-Base-T, FDDI

"store and forward" model. They set up one or more servers on the backbone network. In some cases, this server is capable of accepting any transaction format; it does not have to be HL7, but may be any vendor's record format. This allows both the hospital and the application vendor some breathing room in which to develop the eventual standard transactions. This is a good interim solution but, in the long run, the applications and operating software on each platform will have to be changed.

This achieves horizontal linkages among the business processes. It also can be used to feed multiple transaction processing systems into a consolidated data base for decision support, reporting, and research activities.

Clinical Backbones

Many hospitals are acquiring clinical information systems (CIS) and installing separate clinical backbones to support them. An interesting development is the linking of patient monitor networks to these CIS. Until recently, there has been a clear demarcation between information systems and patient monitoring systems, which display and print various patient physiological data such as pulse, heart rate, CO_2 in blood, temperature, respiration rate, and so on. This has changed. There are now "smart"

Table 6.17 Feasible Health Care Automation Protocol

7	MEDIX, MHS, X.400, FTAM, ROSE, SQL, Windows, SNMP
6	Vendor middleware
5	Vendor middleware
4	TCP, IPX/SPX
3	IP, IPX/SPX
2	802.3, 802.5
1	10-Base-T, FDDI

patient monitors that combine the functionality of both a monitor and a clinical workstation. Monitoring, trending, and reporting can be done from the same device. In addition to displaying and printing the wave forms and values of various parameters, it can also send these (at a hospital-defined frequency) to a Clinical Data Base. For example, it could

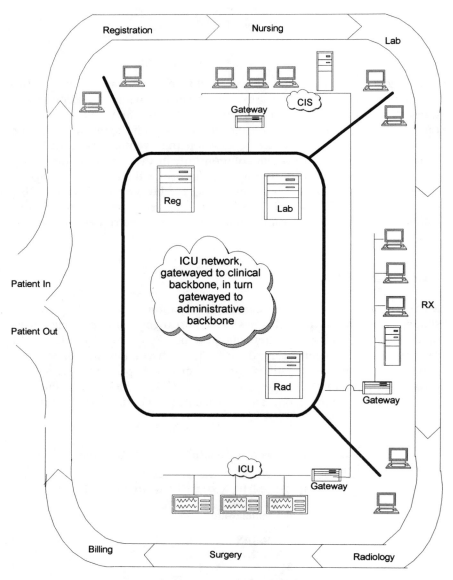

Figure 6.25 Clinical backbone, separate from administrative backbone.

take snapshots of pulse, pressure, respiration, and CO_2 once per second and send them to a patient data base, where they could be compared with norms and care protocols, or they could be used in studies.

Most frequently, the monitors are isolated on a separate ICU network. The traffic is very heavy, and delivery of messages (alarms and ongoing data readouts) for critically ill patients must be guaranteed. This is similar to the needs of process control in manufacturing automation. As in other industries, the same network should not be used both to control an assembly line and to support office automation at the same time. The data is passed to the clinical information system, where it is stored in a data base that integrates all the patient data. Typically, the CIS network is isolated from the backbone HIS network because it receives high volumes of transactions through the monitor gateway. A router is used to segregate HIS transactions that do not have the CIS as their destination. See Figure 6.25.

These clinical information systems present new issues for data base synchronization and data ownership. The registration system owns patient demographic data, but the CIS owns the physiological data. When demographic data changes, should the HIS broadcast to the monitors, or should the HIS broadcast it to the CIS, which in turn alerts the monitors? Conversely, when physiological data changes, how should the CIS broadcast this to all the ancillaries who might be interested in it?

Suddenly, a completely new area of the hospital data model has appeared—the physiological data entities. The size of the patient data base has increased by an order of magnitude. The size of the data model has also grown considerably. These new clinical entities will be joined to financial, physician, and demographic data bases for epidemiological research and analysis of care patterns to determine effectiveness, both for outcomes and costs.

Medical Information Bus

As mentioned above, end users are not the only hospital entities that generate data. The monitoring devices attached to patients are capable of generating data non stop. The OSI model applies to this situation as well. There need to be standards for physical connectivity, for routing of messages, and for the structure of the messages that are sent. The Medical Information Bus (MIB) is an IEEE project to produce these standards. Not only will MIB provide for the automated capture of bedside data into the chart, it will also allow remote/automated adjustment of the devices. The devices include: physiological data monitors, ventilators, IV pumps, and so on. MIB represents process control—the shop floor collection of data. As such, it stands in the same relation to MEDIX as MAP to TOP in the manufacturing industry. MAP stands for Manufacturing Automation Protocol, and TOP stands for Technical Office Protocol. Both of

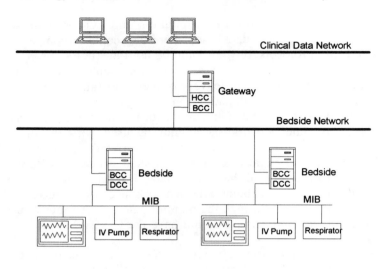

HCC = Clinical Network Connection
BCC = Bedside Communicaations Controller
DCC = Device Communications Controller

Figure 6.26 Medical information bus (MIB).

them are IEEE 7-layer standards. General Motors, for example, uses MAP to connect and control all its shop floor robots. MAP specifies the physical and logical connectivity for these robots. The physical connection is through a deterministic protocol such as Token Ring (or deterministic Ethernet—Ethernet at Level 1 and a deterministic protocol at Level 2). The transactions that keep the network in synchronization are called MMS (= Manufacturing Message System). TOP, on the other hand, is a suite of protocols that support the connection of end-user activities such as electronic mail and file exchange. It uses many of the protocols that we have discussed so far. Unlike MAP, TOP networks do not require a deterministic network, and they frequently run over a contention type of network like Ethernet.

In Figure 6.26 each bed has a controller unit and a mini network of medical devices. The controller takes the data and forwards it onto the monitor network. It may be sent to another monitor, for remote monitoring, or it may be sent through a gateway onto the clinical data network, which is for end users.[5]

---

[5] For an overview of the MIB, see Lorene S. Nolan and M. Michael Shabot, "The P1073 Medical Information Bus Standard: Overview and Benefits for Clinical Users," *Proceedings of the Fourteenth Annual Symposium on Computer Applications in Medical Care* (IEEE Computer Society Press, 1990), pp. 216–219.

7
Control Architecture

The preceding three chapters on architecture dealt with models and methods for aligning a hospital's information systems with its business processes. From time to time, particularly in the "General Discussion" and "Management Discussion" sections, these chapters alluded to the fact that another structure needs to be in place to ensure that the organization actually behaves according to these models. Beyond knowledge of networking protocols and capacity management, there must be an organizational culture that permits this. There has to be some structure to set priorities, to establish and enforce standards, to influence behavior through the right assortment of financial and budgetary incentives, to set and enforce policies, and to ensure integration. This group of concepts is called the Control Architecture. Its relationship to the other architectures is shown in Figure 7.1.

This chapter deals with management issues, not technical issues. This is appropriate, since the Control Architecture is simply the application of general management principles within a technical framework.

Many hospitals, on paper at least, appear to have the components of a Control Architecture in place. There is a Management Engineering department to assist with the design of the business process; there is a Strategic Planning department; there is a backbone network and data management software. In spite of this, a good fit between systems and strategy is missing, as evidenced by the following:

- Multiple departments buy redundant systems.
- Interfaces among systems are inconsistent.
- It is impossible to get an integrated view of data for clinical, financial, or QA purposes.
- End users do not use the system properly.
- Anticipated productivity gains are not achieved.

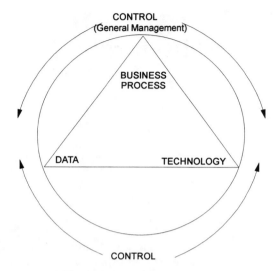

Figure 7.1 Architectures.

- Standards are not observed.
- Insufficient resources are committed to important systems projects.
- Information technology is acquired without consideration of hospital strategy.

Most of the above problems reveal a failure to observe principles of general management. They cannot be attributed to technology. Rather, the problem is with methodology: how existing technology is managed and used. Most information systems failures are not technology failures; they are methodology and management failures. The problems enumerated above show the following problems with general management:

- Failure to assess and manage risk.
- Failure to establish priorities and standards.
- Failure to build organizational consensus and shared vision.
- Failure to establish and enforce policies.
- Failure to empower technical staff with the proper tools, skills, and authority.
- Failure to set goals, measure performance, and follow up.

Traditionally, general management has avoided dealing with information systems issues because of their assumed technical complexity. But one of the megatrends of the 1990s is the pressure on general management to come to grips with the lower levels of the organization, and this includes information technology. Total Quality Management, flattened hierarchies, and business reengineering are causing this megatrend.

Chapters 4 through 6 attempted to provide a technical framework for making management decisions about technical subjects. This chapter discusses the controls that make the architectures work. This idea of a Control Architecture will require fundamental shifts in corporate culture, structure, and skills. However, these are the same changes required by TQM, flattening, and reengineering. The traditional model of corporate management is becoming obsolete. This model is departmentally focused, hierarchical, and distanced from the actual business processes that it is supposed to manage. To a great extent, this management model is formed and reinforced by the Control Architecture of the company. Through its policies and procedures, the Control Architecture defines and rewards behavior according to this model. The Control Architecture can also be used to create new behaviors that bring information systems into closer alignment with business processes.

Control Architecture and Data Processing Eras

The Control Architecture consists of the policies, procedures, methodologies, organizational structures, and standards employed by the hospital in its *general* management of information systems. (There is a different set of methodologies for *technical* management, such as performance analysis, capacity planning, configuration management, etc. This is in the Technical Architecture.)

The Era model (see Table 7.1), which was originally presented in Chapter 3, turns out to be an excellent way to summarize an organization's Control Architecture, using the three categories of administration, user, and justification. (It does not evaluate issues of "fit.") The reader will notice that a fourth era has been added. Many industries have started to build interorganizational systems to support improved operations and strategic partnerships. Such arrangements obviously will require a different Control Architecture. Table 7.2 shows how some of the com-

Table 7.1 Data Processing Eras

	Administration	User	Justification
Era I	Monopoly	Department	Cost/efficiency
Era II	Free market	Individual	Effectiveness
Era III	Regulated free market	Enterprise	Strategic goals
Era IV	Regulated free market *plus* "trade agreement"	Linked enterprises	Mutual strategic goals

Table 7.2 Control Architecture by Era

Era	Characteristics of control architecture
I	The *reward system* is departmental in orientation. No one is encouraged to look beyond departmental boundaries when engaged in problem solving. Projects are *funded* on a departmental basis, and project managers are *rewarded* for bringing the project in under budget and on time. Prioritization is by department. There is little departmental control over the IS *budget*. There are either no *standards* or there are monolithic standards. There is probably no executive systems *steering committee*. The organization has a hierarchical command and control *structure*.
II	The *reward system* is still departmental in orientation. However, new technology gives individuals the opportunity to do their isolated jobs more effectively. Users gain control over their IT *budgets*. If there is an Executive *Steering Committee*, it prioritizes major requests for IT on a departmental basis; for all other requests, it takes a laissez-faire stance. There are no standards. The natural outcome of the hierarchical command and control *structure* is isolation of departments, which go their separate ways in systems development.
III	The *reward system* is driven by contribution to the enterprise as a whole. Departmental needs are suboptimized for the good of the organization. The value system emphasizes the benefits of cooperation and communication. Standards are enforced for technology that impacts the enterprise. Chargebacks and *budgets* are used to achieve IT behaviors that help achieve strategic goals. Prioritization is done through a *steering committee*, and this committee evaluates requests in light of hospital strategy. Strategic planning and systems planning are closely linked. Interdepartmental *structures*, such as teams, are used.
IV	This era has many of the characteristics of Era III, applied to multiple distinct organizations, such as supplier and purchaser. It shows closer collaboration among these entities, such as electronic links between a company and its suppliers, shared data bases, partnerships and joint ventures. This trend has already started, and it requires a control architecture that spans multiple organizations.

ponents of the Control Architecture (reward system, funding system, standards, planning system) work in the various eras.

Despite the trend toward local area networks and PCs, there are still some hospitals that are in Era I. This is not automatically bad, as long as their competitive environment and organizational nature do not demand that they move into Era II or III. However, it is difficult to see how a hospital could remain in this position over time. In reality, most hospitals exhibit characteristics of Era I and Era II simultaneously. For example, a centralized, monopolistic IS department controls the host-based data, while frustrated departments go their own way with their departmental networks and niche systems. This is *not* Era III. Era III has a blending of Eras I and II, not a conflict between them.

Control Architecture and the Seven S's

The Seven S's model, first presented in Chapter 4, illustrates the concept that the components of an organization must "fit" together. It turns out that the Seven S's model is also an effective way to organize and present the components of the Control Architecture. It is useful to review the definition of its categories:

Superordinate Goals: The general goals and values of the organization, together with the mission statement.

Strategy: The business strategies of the hospital. This also includes the information systems strategy.

Structure: The hospital's organizational structure. Is the organization strictly hierarchical, or is there a matrix? Is a particular function centralized or distributed? Where in the hierarchy does a particular function report?

Systems: Both the manual business processes and the automated business processes. A "system" is "how things get done" in a given company. For example, how is Accounts Payable handled? How is budgeting handled? How is prioritization done? What is the measurement and reward system like?

Style: The values, culture, and behavior of hospital management. Is management confrontational or supportive; risk taking or risk averse; empire-building or cooperative; conservative or innovative; insecure or confident?

Staff: Employee positions and job descriptions.

Skills: The skills required by given positions.

Figure 7.2 shows the questions that must be asked when considering a change in strategy. This strategy may not fit with the other components of the company. Either the components must be changed or the strategy must be changed. Table 7.3 examines the components of the Control Architecture by organizing them according to the Seven S's. The most complex areas are Structure and Systems. Structure encompasses all the issues of organizational design that affect the way a hospital uses and manages information systems. Systems refers to all the policies and procedures for doing things that affect information systems: how they are prioritized, how they are funded, how their success is measured, how departmental performance vis-à-vis IS is measured and rewarded.

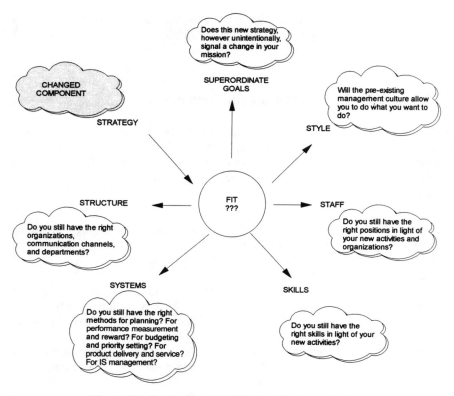

Figure 7.2 Seven S's model for architecture strategy.

One could name many other policies and standards, but they concern the internal operations of the HIS department, not the linkages between systems and business. Examples of this would be policies on systems management and operations (controls, staffing, capacity planning, and configuration management). Whenever a component of the Control Architecture changes, the hospital must evaluate its impact on the other components, as illustrated in Figure 7.3, which shows the structural questions that must be asked when a hospital is considering the adoption of a systems integration strategy.

Variation in Control Architecture

There is no single "ideal" Control Architecture. Some hospitals will show greater centralization of decisions; some hospitals will show greater decentralization of IS. They will differ in how they charge back for IS services. Much of this is driven by Strategy. If the hospital's strategy is

Table 7.3 Aspects of the Seven S's

	Superordinate goals
Corporate culture	Is the culture based on cooperation or confrontation? Do individuals and departments believe that it is a good thing to do what is "right" for the hospital? Is there frequent "suboptimizing," whereby the efficiency of a department is maximized to the detriment of the hospital as a whole? What is the attitude towards consultants?
Tribal knowledge	Do members of top management all have the same paradigm for how systems articulate with strategy and business processes? What is their world view? Does management understand methodologies such as accounting, public relations and marketing, departmental management, budgeting, and business planning? Is there a broad understanding among employees of what the hospital stands for, what its mission is, how its business processes fit together? Do consulting engagements achieve the appropriate knowledge transfer?
	Strategy
Vision	Does the strategic plan result in a strategic vision and a systems vision?
Architecture	Is the tribal knowledge reinforced through documentation of the architectures? Are the architectures maintained? Are they enforced? Do they fit together?
	Structure
Placement of the IS executive	To whom does the head of IS report—the CEO, CFO, COO? What is the attitude of senior management towards information systems? Does the head of information systems participate with senior management in strategic planning?
Strategic planning function	Is this process centralized and bureaucratic? What do people do with the plan once it has been published? Is it a visible part of management discussions? Does it include an information systems plan? Is the plan understood by top management and by the people who have to implement it? Is it viewed as a working document? Is it developed by the people who will implement it?
Steering committee	Is there a group of executives that meets regularly to decide system priorities and allocate scarce system resources? Do they prioritize based on a plan? Do they understand the issues sufficiently in order to make informed decisions?
Placement of IS resources	How much contact does the IS development staff have with end users? Do development personnel actually work for end-user departments? What IS functions do end-users perform?
Lateral communication and coordination	What are the types and numbers of forums and communications channels whose purpose is to keep the end-user community informed of systems events and decisions? Is continuity ensured by having the same people sit on multiple committees?

(*Continued*)

Table 7.3 *Continued*

Systems	
Centralization versus distribution	Does the hospital have policies for the placement of systems activities such as operations, support, and development? Is it all centralized, or all decentralized? How is systems support performed? Are end users allowed to develop their systems? What types of systems can they develop? Can they change the state of centralized data bases through their self-developed systems? Are there standards for the use of a systems development methodology? How is quality assurance performed, particularly for end-user-developed systems?
Standards development and enforcement	Do standards flow from the architectures? Is there a standard for data modeling, for problem definition, and for analysis? Are there network standards: network operating system, network communications, type of wiring, etc.? Are there standards for SDM deliverables? For hardware and applications software? For data base systems? For when a DBMS should be used? Are there standards for workstations?
Cost/benefit analysis	How are costs and benefits compared? Are the benefits maximized for the short-term only? Is any attention paid to "soft" benefits that are more difficult to quantify? Is there pragmatism, or insistence on system hygiene in every project?
Performance measurement and reward	Are there measures of success for the systems that get implemented? Is there a system of reward and recognition that encourages people to see the broad picture? Are project managers mechanically held to their departmental budgets and time frames? Are TQM principles applied when measuring performance?
Funding of information systems	Who pays for information systems development and support? How is the Information Systems department set up: as a cost center or as a profit center? Has the organization defined what behaviors it wants to encourage through a chargeback system? If Information Systems is a profit center, does this cause behavior that maximizes the performance of the IS department, but suboptimizes the performance of the organization as a whole? How does the organization motivate users to follow standards in systems selection? How does it discourage the use of older, less efficient systems?
Information systems development	Is there a documented SDM? Do the information systems people understand how to use it, and why? Do the end users understand it? Can it be tailored by type of project: end user vs. system professional? Can it be used for either prototyping or straight-line development? Are there well-documented examples of deliverables?
Feasibility and project initiation	Does the organization require an initial analysis to determine project feasibility? Is this analysis tied to the plan? What role does the Steering Committee play in this?

(Continued)

Table 7.3 *Continued*

Systems	
Project management	Do the systems professionals and end users understand project management? Do end users participate in projects? Are there policies for when an end user may be a project leader?
Quality assurance	How is QA performed on systems—as they are developed? After they are developed? What is done to ensure that QA is perceived as a facilitator, not as an obstacle?

Style	
Management attitudes and behavior	Does management say one thing and do another? Does it punish failure? Does it promote common goals?

Staff	
Job positions	Management of systems architecture as described in this book will require new skills and jobs. Is there a Data Administration function and position? Is there a Standards function and position? Is there an integration function and position?

Skills	
Skills within positions	Do managers understand how to do organization of redesign and write job descriptions? Do systems developers have integration skills as well as communication skills? Are end users, both staff and management, regularly educated about IS issues and trends?

heavily geared toward independent product lines, and the profit strategy is to maximize each department by letting them compete against each other, then one type of control architecture would be more appropriate than another.

The "ultimate" critera for the goodness of the Control Architecture are the degree of alignment of the information systems with the business architecture, the success of IS projects, and the concomitant success of the company. Given the diversity among hospitals, the eventual form assumed by the Control Architecture in a given hospital will be influenced by many things: size, resources, mission, competitive environment, strategy, geographical area, and so forth.

In general, hospitals that are exclusively in Era I or Era II are dysfunctional. Era III represents a balance between IS control of information systems and end-user control. The range of acceptable balance is shown in Figure 7.4. The current health care environment (and the rest of the 1990s) requires hospitals to change, to reengineer their business processes and align systems with these processes. Era I Control Architecture is too

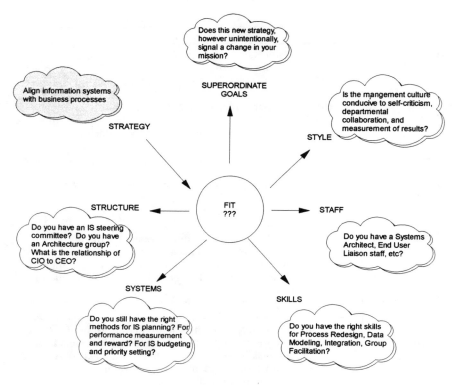

Figure 7.3 Seven S's model.

rigid to allow change. Era II controls are too chaotic to permit an organized approach to problem solving.

It is difficult to quantify the metrics for centralization and decentralization. They are shown descriptively in Figure 7.5. Several representative components of the Control Architecture have been plotted, each on its own axis. Along any axis, the closer one gets to the center, the greater the amount of Era I control (centralization). The closer to the periphery, the greater the amount of Era II control (decentralization). The dot indicates an even balance of the particular component. The shaded area represents the range of acceptable variation for each component. As long as a hospital "profile" is within this shaded area, one can say that there is an acceptable fit between the Control Architecture and the information systems. Figure 7.6 contrasts two hospitals: one is within the acceptable range of variation; the other has several components that are outside this range.

Hospital A displays a Reward System and Budgeting System that are not very close to the ideal norm, but which still are within the acceptable

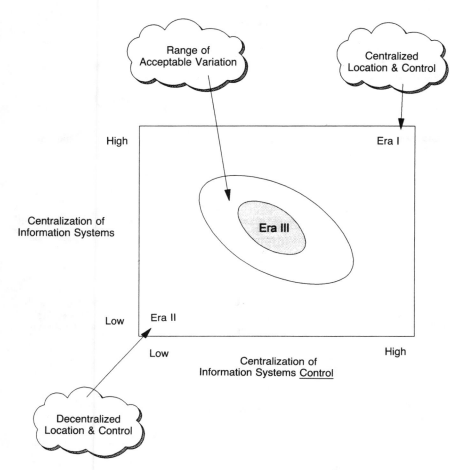

Figure 7.4 DP eras and control architecture variation.

range. Hospital B, on the other hand, has several components that are outside this range (Management Control and Reward System). Hospital B insists on doing strategic planning for systems in a fairly centralized fashion, but much of the systems management is done on a locally decentralized basis. The latter is encouraged by a reward system which is departmentally oriented. IS budgets are mutually developed, but there is no control over how they are spent. There is a steering committee that is out of touch with the departments. If the business strategy requires close cooperation among business processes (and thus linkages among systems), it will be frustrated.

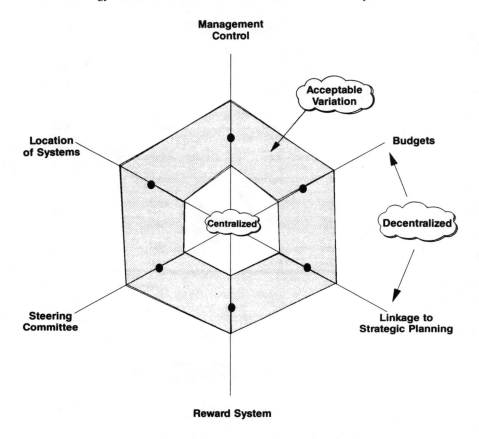

Figure 7.5 Range of variation of control architecture.

Control Architecture and Organizational Type

This last section examines potential variations in the Control Architecture of four different hospitals: (1) a chain, (2) a public hospital, (3) a teaching hospital, (4) a community hospital.

Hospital Chain: This is a diverse group of hospitals, ranging from traditional private-pay, indemnity-based hospitals to HMOS (see Table 7.4).
Public Hospital: These are hospitals chartered and funded by governmental agencies (federal, state, city, county, et al.). See Table 7.5.
Teaching Hospital: Hospitals affiliated with a medical school (see Table 7.6).

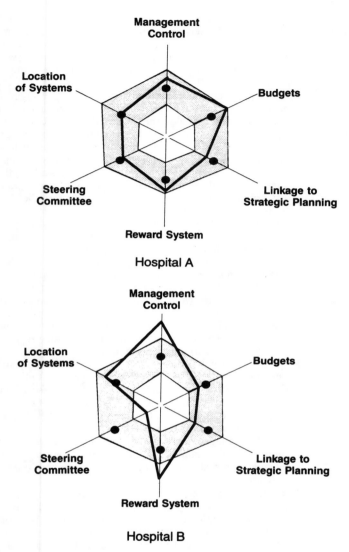

Figure 7.6 Comparison of two hospitals' control architectures.

Community Hospital: Typically, the stand-alone, adult critical-care hospital. This is also a very diverse group of hospitals, ranging from the indemnity-based model to the HMO model (see Table 7.7).

This approach could be applied to group practices and the other provider entities that have appeared in recent years.

Table 7.4 Seven S's for Hospital Chain

	Hospital chain
Superordinate goals	A chain can be either for-profit or not-for-profit. Superordinate goals are usually fairly simple: Provide quality care and a return to investors (if for-profit). Chains that grow by acquisition or merger have problems creating a common culture.
Strategy	Chains can have widely varying business strategies regarding products, markets, image, etc. They can also have different IT strategies, depending on the desired degree of corporate control. Information systems can be used to enforce control, to differentiate hospitals, to build a national image, or to keep patients within the hospital chain. The basic decision is: Does the company need tight integration of systems across the enterprise, or does the corporate headquarters function more as a holding company, which requires only periodic transmission of summary data?
	Dichotomy between corporate and local hospitals.
	• The corporate strategy might be to function as a holding company, requiring a predefined rate of return from each hospital, but otherwise not interfering. In this case, the corporation needs minimal amounts of data from its hospitals. Each hospital has a strategy based on local competitive conditions, which would entail different information systems strategies. One hospital may be the low-cost provider. Another might pursue value-added, through information systems. If local strategies are all different, then it is difficult for corporations to impose standards.
	• On the other hand, the chain might decide that corporate headquarters can provide centralized expertise to the decentralized hospitals, in areas such as purchasing, materials management, management engineering, JCAHO preparation, and HCFA relations. Or, they may desire to develop a national image. In this case, corporate strategy requires more data for management, requiring much tighter systems integration and standardization. Corporate strategy might even decide to have large centralized systems for use by individual hospitals.
Structure	The issues of organizational structure are numerous and complex: steering committees, the existence and placement of a CIO, the location of IS department(s), the location of user-support groups, the structure of IS project teams, etc. (The same issues face each of the traditional "functional" areas: Finance, Marketing, etc.) This can be further complicated by the existence of regional administrations.
	• A chain is likely to have a CIO position at corporate headquarters, with IS directors in the local hospitals. However, the degree to which this person actually functions as a CIO—linking business and systems strategy and then enforcing these linkages—depends on whether the corporation interferes with the strategy and operations of its member hospitals. A lack of fit would occur where the hospital has its own specific systems while corporate headquarters is overly concerned with enforcing corporate standards for hospital-internal networks.
	• In a chain, it is unlikely that the local hospitals will have significant IS operations outside of HIS, while in other types

(Continued)

Table 7.4 *Continued*

Hospital chain

	of hospitals, particularly teaching hospitals, this is frequently the case.
	• In a centralized approach, the steering committee will have to be drawn from the hospitals in the chain. In a decentralized approach, each hospital will already have a committee, formed from administrators within the hospital.
	• If a chain centralizes its development and operations it must be careful not to overcentralize the support functions. If the help desk, training, and hardware support are remote, users will underutilize the system and look for alternate systems that they can acquire for themselves.
	• In a centralized approach, one still needs to get user buy-in and ownership of the systems. This is accomplished by user groups. The roll-out of common systems can be problematic. How does one assemble a team of systems people for local installation when the local hospital has a "lights out" approach to systems?
Systems	The term "system" refers to the ways in which things get done in the organization; it includes "reward system," "budgeting system," and "planning system." In a chain, some systems are more extensive than in stand-alone hospitals. For example, Materials Management (inventory control, purchasing, receiving, accounts payable) might be done on a corporate-wide basis. Standards development, education, and enforcement can be greatly complicated by the chain's multiple locations. Problems with fit occur when there is a corporate standard, but the reward systems of each hospital do not agree with it. For example, does one circumvent the Materials Management controls because management wants to order a nonstandard item? Or, in another case, the budgeting system does not allow for differences in hospital-level strategy.
	A problem can occur when a corporate strategy of common systems clashes with a reward system based solely on individual hospital performance.
Style	Each local hospital is likely to have its own corporate culture, particularly when the chain grows by acquisition. Information systems can assist in creating a common culture, since they can provide organizational feedback as well as financial feedback (through teleconferencing, Email, or shared data bases). Or, if the chain is trying to build a national image, local differences in corporate culture could militate against this. Local differences could also prevent integration of existing systems. There can be conflicts between the corporate bureaucracy and the entrepreneurial local hospital.
Staff	Regardless of the degree of centralization or decentralization, a chain has great need for positions that do communication and coordination across the chain.
Skills	A chain that owns small hospitals, particularly in urban areas, will have difficulty attracting and retaining systems personnel. If its systems strategy requires significant skills at the local level, how will it achieve this? If a higher degree of control is desired, together with local autonomy in system selection, what kinds of positions need to be defined in order to ensure data integration, conformance to standards, education?

(Continued)

Table 7.4 *Continued*

Hospital chain
If corporate IS staff will be doing significant development for local hospitals, how do they ensure communication and coordination with the hospitals in the field? How does one ensure the maintenance of local computer skills when there is a remote centralized support staff, in the face of 15–20% local staff turnover?

Table 7.5 Seven S's for Public Hospital

	Public hospital
Superordinate goals	On paper it has a relatively simple mission: to provide quality care to those who cannot afford it and to provide emergency care. Some of them are connected with medical schools, and this complicates their mission (see comments on Teaching Hospitals).
Strategy	A consistent, long-range business strategy is difficult to formulate, since the hospital is frequently driven by the political expediencies of the govermental agency that oversees it. Thus, there is probably little linkage between general strategy and systems strategy. A generic strategy of high value-added does not make sense, so the de facto strategy is mass-market low-cost producer. In a sense, these hospitals have a captive market segment for which no one else is competing. Thus there is little external motivation to have an architected approach to systems management.
Structure	The head of information systems, even if he is called a CIO, probably reports to a financial officer (particularly in stand-alone hospitals). There is a single, centralized IS department. Public hospitals can have multiple locations, such as countywide. In this case coordination of systems could become more complicated. Hierarchical structures predominate, with little lateral coordination.
Systems	The business processes are highly bureaucratic and politicized. The reward system is the classical governmental one: length of service and political connection; and there is probably no performance measurement. The system for prioritization of IT requests does not take the enterprise view. The actual information systems are unlikely to be open, with the possible exception of federal systems, which require that purchases conform to the OSI standards. The budgeting system is top-down and departmentally oriented.
Style	Corporate culture is likely to be risk-averse, buck-passing, conservative, department oriented rather than enterprise oriented and entrepreneurial. Innovation is not encouraged.
Staff	Because of the extremely cost-oriented environment, little attention is likely to be paid to long-term staff needs, or to positions such as systems planners or data administrators.
Skills	Skills are likely to be insufficient, except in those community hospitals that are teaching hospitals.

Table 7.6 Seven S's for Teaching Hospital

	Teaching hospital
Superordinate goals	Its mission is likely to be more complex—a combination of patient care, teaching, and research, with heavy emphasis on charity care and community service and leadership. Almost universally not-for-profit (it is impossible to maintain such high staff-patient ratios in an investor-owned environment), these hospitals tend to be urban.
Strategy	Development of a coherent strategy can be hindered by the large number of diverse and powerful stakeholders: hospital administration, medical school administration, doctors, board of trustees, public agencies, etc. If it is decided to link systems strategy with business strategy, the effort is very complicated because of the addition of teaching and research.
Structure	Management structure is likely to be very complicated. There are two powerful hierarchies, administrative and medical staff, resulting in complex matrix management. While the administrative model is centralized and bureaucratic, each clinical department is very powerful, resulting in multiple bureaucracies. Influential medical school departments are likely to have their own sophisticated systems and systems organizations (e.g., Laboratory, Radiology, Surgery). It can be difficult to assemble and effectively manage a steering committee for IT prioritization. As a result, it can be difficult to define and enforce standards for enterprise computing. Their data needs are more complicated than other hospitals. A CIO at the level of the CFO and COO is very common.
Systems	The complex, conservative organizational structure is reflected in the systems for funding, standards-setting, rewarding, planning, priortization, and others.
Style	Forming a consistent corporate culture often proves to be difficult. The culture of physicians is very different from that of administrators. Because of their rigorous training and work environment, physicians frequently exhibit machismo, and this is antithetical to a culture of cooperation. The self-perception of omnipotence can prevent empowerment of other staff.
Staff	This type of hospital is likely to have abundant resources of IT. Many of the departments connected with the medical school might have their own systems, which they run, support, and develop.
Skills	There is likely to be a very high level of technical skills. This is offset by the extremely difficult nature of communications and coordination.

Table 7.7 Seven S's for Community Hospital

	Community hospital
Superordinate goals	These hospitals are quite diverse. They may be for-profit or not-for-profit. They may be urban or suburban. (For purposes of exposition, rural hospitals are excluded, and teaching hospitals were discussed separately.) There is great variance in size, which impacts their ability to do things with information technology.
Strategy	These hospitals feel the effects of competition much more than the teaching hospitals and public hospitals, and so they are looking for strategies to differentiate themselves and to lock in patients and doctors. Thus, they have a strong motivation to link systems planning with business planning. Some of these hospitals are doctor-owned, the strategy being to lock in the referrals. Many of them seek to be "niche" providers, concentrating on one or two services. This would indicate a need for niche information services to differentiate them.
Structure	Management structure is fairly centralized and simple. While it is a hierarchy, it is fairly flat, with a CEO, COO, CFO, and few other top level managers such as vice presidents. The IS department is centralized, and most frequently reports to the CFO. This depends on the size of the hospital and the personality of the CEO. The larger hospitals are more likely to have a CIO. In others, the CEO has taken a personal interest in the use of technology.
Systems	Community hospitals have simpler systems for funding, standards-setting, rewarding, planning, and prioritization. In theory, this should permit the shift to an architected approach to information systems. Resources, however, can be a problem.
Style	This situation is more conducive to building a consistent culture. Community hospitals do not have the diversity of a chain or a teaching hospital. Small size is a mixed blessing. The hospital in theory can move faster and with greater coordination. However, there are fewer resources available to do this.
Staff	A big problem is resources—many individuals will have to perform multiple functions.
Skills	IT skills are likely to be lower than in other types of hospitals. This is offset by the fact that the computer systems are more likely to be less heterogeneous than in other environments. However, there is an industry trend to consolidation and electronic linkages among organizations (hospitals, payers, regulators, government, physicians, suppliers, etc.). This will require skills and resouces, which otherwise would not be needed to run the information systems.

8
Abbreviated Methodology

Chapter 8 outlines a methodology for developing the architectures discussed in Chapters 4 through 7. This methodology assumes that a hospital is in Era III for its information systems management, and is high-high on the strategic grid (Figure 8.1). The reader will recall that Era III is marked by a balance among IS, end users, and top executives in the management of information technology. Most hospitals are located in the high-high quadrant of the strategic grid, depending heavily on information systems support of product delivery and marketing. There may be some hospitals that are not high-high on the strategic grid. Such hospitals might include small single-provider rural hospitals.

This methodology is only an outline, not a substitute for the many full-blown planning methodologies offered by consultants and vendors. These include generic cross-industry methodologies, such as Business Systems Planning (IBM), Method One (Andersen Consulting), and Information Engineering (Ernst and Young). Firms that specialize in health care consulting, such as Sheldon Dorenfest and Associates, JDA, or First Consulting, have their own methodologies.

The complexity of systems integration and process redesign, together with flattening and outsourcing, will force both general managers and technical managers to turn to third parties for help. The intent of this chapter is to provide a framework for the hospital to evaluate the proposals and activities of both consultants and vendors. While each third-party planning methodology employs a somewhat different terminology, they all involve the same basic steps and they all produce equivalent outputs. This book builds on a generic planning methodology and adds the following: four architectures as deliverables (Business, Data, Technical, and Control), the Data Architecture as the principal integrating tool; insistence on business process redesign; and insistence that the architec-

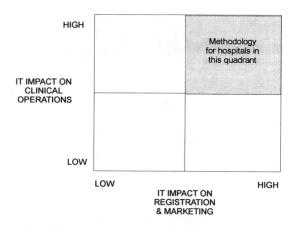

Figure 8.1 Strategic grid.

tural outputs be maintainable and usable as "tribal" knowledge. The thoughtful reader will have noticed that the Control Architecture impacts all systems-related methodologies. As a matter of fact, the successful use of these third-party methodologies depends more on Control Architecture issues than on the inherent goodness of these methodologies.

The methodology outlined in this chapter is also not for systems development or installation. Vendors and consultants can provide the latter. On the Systems Management side there is a large set of well-defined disciplines that are outside the scope of this book. They include: capacity planning, change control, configuration management, systems development, operations management, project management, and end-user support. Obviously, they too depend critically on the Control Architecture.

There are three obstacles to the use of a methodology: culture, skills, and manpower. A hospital needs to know *why* it is bringing in a third-party to develop its architecture. Is it because the hospital has a culture that does not like to "think" or does not like to take responsibility? If so, then methodologies are of no relevance. Hospitals frequently lack the manpower required to perform all the tasks of a project, and so it is quite appropriate to use outside resources. The challenge is for the hospital to maintain a core group of in-house personnel with the skills necessary to manage the consultants. If there will be a chronic shortage of manpower, it is critical to have these in-house linkages. Moreover, the hospital must have a management culture that demands accountability of consultants: They must define how they will achieve transfer of any new knowledge to the internal staff, and how this will be measured.

Methodology

There are two major phases: Business Strategy and Systems Strategy (which includes Systems Architecture).

Develop Business Strategy

Guidelines for developing a business strategy are widely known and well documented. The steps include analyzing social, political, and economic trends; assessing the hospital's strengths and weaknesses, particularly in comparison with competitors; and prioritizing the major issues that it must address to survive over time, so that it can fulfill its mission. This is summarized in Figure 8.2.

It is worthwhile to review the steps for formulating the general business strategy, since this process produces outputs that can be used in the formulation of the four architectures and the general IT strategy; conversely, this process can use the outputs of the architectures. For example, when evaluating the internal environment it can be useful to have documentation of the current business processes.

Each step in Figure 8.2 has a shadow activity, which represents the parallel activity for Information Systems. While some staff are assembling data on the external economic environment, others may be doing the same thing for technology trends. In this way, the hospital develops its IT strategy at the same time as its business strategy, and thus IT can influence the business strategy while the latter is still being formulated. The details of these "shadow" IT activities will be discussed later.

1. *Assess the External Environment*: This is the information-gathering stage. The hospital collects data on its industry and the broader external environment. The data to be collected includes economic trends, social issues, political issues, demographics, competitor performance and actions. This also includes analysis of the industry structure: the relative strength of suppliers and customers, distribution channels, and so on.

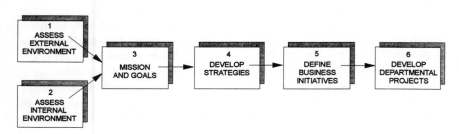

Figure 8.2 Strategic planning model.

At the national level, much data is available from the U.S. government, the AHA, and consulting firms. At the local level, the hospital will have to do its own data gathering. The AHA publishes an excellent guide on how to perform an assessment.

2. *Assess the Internal Environment*: The hospital reviews its performance, expressed both qualitatively and quantitatively. Performance indicators include financial ratios, market share, turnover ratios, costs, surveys, trends, and quality indicators. It is also important to compare these indicators against those of peers and/or competitors. This step also examines the hospital's strengths and weaknesses. An important element in this is a Seven S's analysis. What has gone right and why? Where has there been a good fit? Where has there not been a good fit? An important result of this is to build the "tribal knowledge" of hospital employees. The internal assessment should be done in a non-accusatory, fact-based fashion, to maximize analysis and minimize insecurity. This should be done with the participation of the managers whose areas are being analyzed.

Consulting firms may be used to perform this assessment. The problem is that much of their analysis will be self-serving. One possible solution is to have this work reviewed by another consultant. Another solution is to maintain staff who are qualified to review the consultants.

3. *Mission and Goals*: The hospital reaffirms its identity, values and goals. Were previous goals realistic? Are new goals necessary? What does the organization believe in and how is that demonstrated by management? What is the mission? During the 1980s, some hospitals may have veered from their mission, as they set up nonhospital subsidiaries to make up for reduced revenues from patient care. During the 1990s, some hospitals will broaden their mission in geographical terms; others may see social issues that cause them to broaden their mission to include education and preventive medicine.

It can be very valuable to use an external consultant. This person provides objectivity and has no history with the participants.

4. *Develop Strategies*: Using what has been learned about the external environment, its internal skills, and its mission and goals, the hospital then develops a set of strategies that will allow it to achieve its long-range goals. Subsequently, the strategies will be converted into concrete business initiatives, and then into projects at the departmental level. Strategies may require the hospital to change existing systems and organizations. Strategy formulation is done through a combination of brainstorming, analysis, and group consensus activities. It may require multiple iterations. It can be very valuable to enlist the help of a consultant to go through different types of planning exercises, "what-if" analysis, SWOT analysis, brainstorming, and so on.

5. *Define Business Initiatives*: These are the projects and programs used to realize new strategies or to continue existing strategies. Even-

tually, these initiatives will be implemented as a series of projects and events at the department level. Some initiatives address business "infrastructure" issues, such as the recruitment and retention of qualified staff; others deal with new programs and clinical services. Some initiatives concern elements of the Control Architecture, such as a project to set up a prioritization process for information systems projects.

6. *Develop Departmental Plans*: Eventually, the initiatives become a project for one or more departments. At the department level, strategic thinking means aligning departmental objectives with hospital objectives and developing plans for their attainment.

The planning process does not have to be a burden. Once the process has been formally initiated, the plan can be incrementally modified each year, or on some cyclical basis. The real challenge is to produce something that can be easily understood, easily modified, and straightforwardly implemented and measured. For this reason, it is important to produce a plan at several levels: (1) the strategic plan; (2) the systems plan and financial plan; (3) departmental plans and budgets. People who will implement the plan must be involved with its production.

The flow of the activities presented in Figure 8.2 can be somewhat misleading—it seems to imply that the process is linear. In actuality, the process is iterative. As strategies are developed, the mission statement may need to be reexamined; as business intitiatives are defined, strategies may need to be reevaluated.

Develop Business Strategy: Deliverables

What is important is that, at the end of the process, the hospital has a set of documents that encapsulate the knowledge gained during the planning process, and which are available as a common resource. Figure 8.3 shows them as outputs of the process. Table 8.1 presents a brief commentary on them.

Develop Systems Strategy

Figure 8.4 shows the cycle for developing an information systems strategy. The blank boxes behind the shaded ones represent the parallel activities for developing the Business Plan. They interact with the systems-related activities. Like business strategic planning, the activities for developing a systems strategy are overlapping and iterative. And, in actuality, some of these activities go on continuously. For example, technology assessment might be done on a year-round basis.

1. *Assess Technology Trends*: This is similar to assessing the external business environment. The hospital collects data on technology trends.

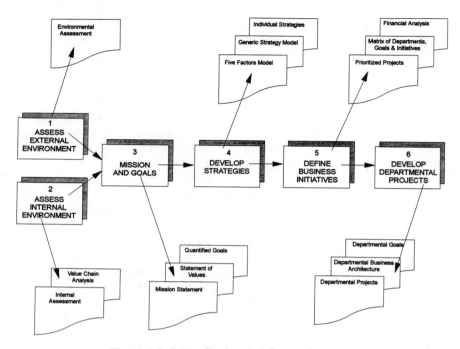

Figure 8.3 Strategic planning flow and outputs.

Which technologies are purely developmental, which are proven? What is the business case for a given technology, and which hospital business processes could it benefit? The hospital must also determine which vendors are stable. What are the competitors doing in the area of systems? What are the trends in information systems management and development? There are several good sources for this data: industry-specific publications, general publications on information systems, consultants, and peer hospitals.

2. *Assess Internal Use of Technology*: The hospital evaluates its information systems and its personnel, using service-level indicators such as response time, uptime, elapsed time to answer a call to the Help Desk, variances from budgeted expenses, project on-time completion rates, user satisfaction, and so forth. If it does not have such measures, it should establish them. Based on existing goals, does the HIS organization have the appropriate skills and structure? Recall what was said about the Seven S's in Chapter 7. Is there a fit? The existing information systems constitute a portfolio that must be evaluated for age, stability, functionality, and architecture. Does the architecture fit the business environment? Are the systems used effectively? Does staff have the correct attitude/values for its functions? What is the size of the HIS budget, and how does it compare to that of competitors/peers?

3. *Mission and Goals*: Working with hospital management, the HIS department defines its own goals, mission, and identity. The HIS department is like a business within a business. What is the role of the HIS department—strategic, support? Should it make a profit? Who are its customers? What Era is it in? Is there a fit between the strategy and the structure or staff? If the hospital's competitive situation has changed, then it may be appropriate to change the goals of the HIS department. For example, the hospital may decide that the IS department should adopt the role of a change agent, actively suggesting technology-based improvements in the value chain and helping to reengineer business processes.

4. *Develop IT Strategies*: Using what has been learned so far in the IT planning process, and combining it with outputs from the business strategy process, the HIS department defines its strategy and architecture. For strategy, the following issues are decided: What is the approach to systems development: build or buy? What is the approach to systems management: centralized or decentralized? What is the approach to the use of new technologies: first mover or early adopter? To what degree should systems be aligned with business processes? What is the approach to technical staff: outside consultants or internal staff? To what extent should the end user be involved with development? What will be the method for development?

This activity includes definition of the four Architectures. This is the conceptual level of the systems architecture, and does not include the implementation-specific details. It takes the important business processes from the strategy/initiatives and creates a high-level design of how information systems should be aligned. The architecture statement might also include the systems vision.

For a hospital that is just beginning to formalize its architectures, much work has to be done defining policy and procedures and standards. After the architectures have been initially defined, the level of activity drops off. The details of the architectures are filled in through "infrastructure" projects. This phase could also include a high-level timetable for the phased implementation of the architecture.

5. *Define IT Initiatives*: The HIS department defines infrastructure initiatives needed to implement the strategy and architecture. These eventually become projects for one or more departments. What things must the IS do to implement the strategy? This would include activities such as upgrading the data center; and installation of backbone networks, data base tools, application interfaces, and operating systems. On the policy side, it includes the development of methodologies and standards. Some of the IT initiatives will be developed jointly with general management, as the hospital defines the general business initiatives. As more is learned in this phase, the four architectures are modified.

6. *Define Departmental Projects*: HIS projects result from both HIS infrastructure initiatives and end-user initiatives. An end-user project

Table 8.1 Outputs of the Strategy Process

Activity	Deliverable	Comment
Assess external environment	Environmental assessment	This document is the first step in building the "tribal knowledge." However, competitor analysis and internal assessment are more critical.
Assess internal environment	Trending of key indicators	This should include more than financial indicators. It should also include comparison with competitors.
	Value chain analysis	This is a high-level value chain. The high-level indicators show variances, but with no explanations. It is the first step in the detailed problem analysis that will follow. Typically, value chain analysis is not performed.
Mission and goals	Mission statement	This is necessary to provide direction and scope. It should not be longer than 4–5 sentences. It should be reviewed periodically, to determine whether changes in the environment dictate a need to change the mission statement, or to determine whether the hospital might be moving in a direction that is outside the scope of its mission.
	Statement of values	Useful when defining architectures. The values of the organization will shape the Control Architecture.
	Quantified goals	In order to determine whether the accomplishment of the mission can be measured, the hospital has to set long-range goals. Later, when budgets are being developed, these are translated into departmental goals/objectives.
Define strategies	Five Factors model	This is a means to an end. It facilitates communication, sets the context, and sets the stage for further analysis.
	Generic Strategy model	This serves the same purpose as Five Factors.
	Strategies	The hospital should have 4–6 strategies. They should not be so narrow that they define projects; they should not be so broad, that they are unimplementable. An effective way to structure the statement of a strategy is the following: In light of . . . . (situation) The hospital will . . . . (action) By . . . . (how, where, etc.) With the result that . . . . (measures)
Develop business initiatives	Prioritized projects	Some of these will be infrastructure projects, such as setting up elements of the Control Architecture (steering committee, reward system, system for priority setting).

(Continued)

Table 8.1 *Continued*

Activity	Deliverable	Comment
	Matrix of departments, goals, and initiatives	The major projects and directions are set by administration; when doing its annual budget, each department aligns its activities with the hospital's goals.
	Financial analysis	The financial plan.
Develop departmental plans	Budgets and plans	Each initiative results in one or more projects at the departmental level.

could be the acquisition of a new Radiology information system. An infrastructure project could include staff, facilities, policies, and computing infrastructure such as a network, data base management system, and so on. It could also include a project for the Systems Development organization to write a methodology to be incorporated into the Control Architecture. As a matter of fact, many organizations do a very poor job of project initiation. The do not have a method for developing and reviewing a feasibilty package, which would contain analysis of costs and benefits, and how the proposed system would fit into the Technical Architecture. This is another aspect of the Control Architecture, and it shows how profoundly general management principles affect information systems.

Architectures

The Architectures (Business, Data, Technical, and Control) are built incrementally, with each iteration of the planning process. It is not likely that a hospital could develop them with one "big bang" in one iteration of the planning cycle. This is an ongoing process. The first round of architectural work will be difficult. Each year, as more is learned about technology, hospital performance, and strategy, it is upgraded. The IS department should not, indeed cannot, develop these architectures alone.

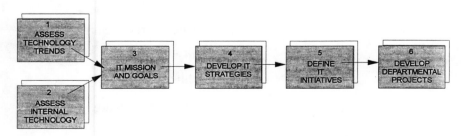

Figure 8.4 IS strategy model.

The Business Architecture is developed primarily by end-user departments. The Control Architecture is decided upon by general management,
using HIS as the design consultant. IS and the end users together develop
the Data Architecture. IS is primarily responsible for developing the
Technical Architecture. Figure 8.5 shows how the architectures are developed incrementally and with input from the non-HIS organizations.
Figure 8.6 shows the outputs of each activity.

Control Architecture: This is only partially the domain of the Information Systems department. Most of the critical decisions concerning
controls must be made by executive management. HIS can design the
controls, but top management must understand and approve them.
Much of the Control Architecture concerns the hospital's organizational structure and policies: how it budgets, prioritizes, solves problems,
and so on. Some of its elements are best decided by HIS—the choice of
a development methodology, for example. However, policies concerning the enforcement of the methodology's use are the purview of
management. If the Control Architecture is not appropriate, or if it is
not enforced, then attempts at building the other architectures will fail.
All Control Architecture projects are infrastructure projects. The
Control Architecture also changes over time, but it changes more
slowly than the business and technical architectures.

Business Architecture: This activity is only partially the responsibility of
the Information Systems department. Primary responsibility belongs to
the user departments. HIS assists departments to define the Business

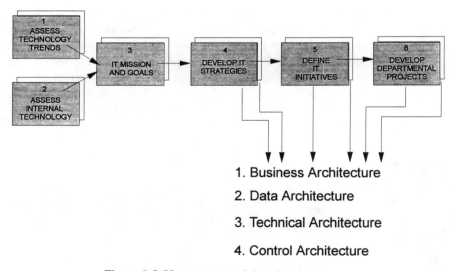

1. Business Architecture

2. Data Architecture

3. Technical Architecture

4. Control Architecture

Figure 8.5 IS strategy model and architectures.

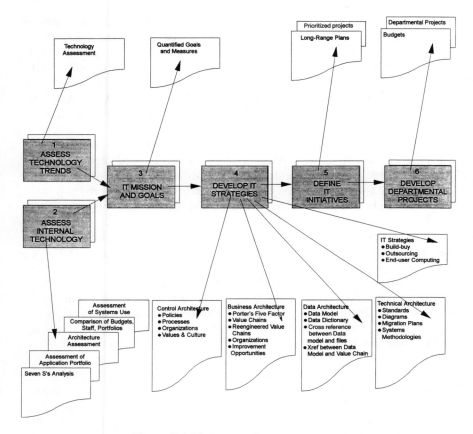

Figure 8.6 IS strategy flow and outputs.

Architecture in the course of a systems development project. The Business Architecture is critical because most decisions to acquire an information system are driven by dissatisfaction with the existing business processes. However, if the hospital does not have a Business Architecture, it focuses on technology, and business process redesign, if it is done at all, is done only after the installation of the information system.

Another source for the Business Architecture is the analysis that is done when the hospital is assessing its internal environment and defining business initiatives. It results from work done to understand the value chains of the major business processes. Finally, the Business Architecture components should flow from a department's commitment to Total Quality Management. If application of TQM principles does not produce that level of analysis, then it is not TQM.

Data Architecture: The Information Systems department is primarily responsible for the Data Architecture, but cannot develop it without the cooperation of end-user departments. The Data Architecture gets built as part of the systems development activity, and as part of the HIS infrastructure activity. The Data Architecture can be developed in parallel with the Business Architecture. However, the Data Architecture cannot be completed until the Business Architecture is finished.

The major component of the Data Achitecture is the Data Model. It provides the key to logical integration of multiple systems, and it plays an important role in requirements definition projects. It provides a Rosetta stone for HIS staff who need to communicate with general management and end users. Over time, the Data Model changes as the competitive environment changes.

Data modeling skills are lacking in most hospitals. Consultants can be useful for installing a methodology and training internal staff.

Technical Architecture: The IS department has primary responsibility for the Technical Architecture, and does all the work on it. The Technical Architecture gets defined in the following ways: (1) through the systems development process, as new aspects of the Business Architecture become known; and (2) through the HIS infrastructure process. The Technical Architecture changes over time, and some aspects of it can change quickly and often, like cabling standards. This change, however, merely underscores the need for the Technical Architecture.

It should be emphasized that the creation of the Technical Architecture is an iterative process. On an ongoing basis, the hospital reviews those cases where the Technical Architecture is not aligned with the Business and Data Architectures, and it judges the economic and technical feasibility of bringing it into alignment.

Develop Systems Strategy: Deliverables

Table 8.2 provides further commentary on the outputs of this activity.

Sample Outputs

Each of the four architectures has a variety of documents. Some are diagramatic (Data Model, value chains); others are textual (policies and procedures). Some are analytical (value chain); others are normative (standards). Some are highly technical; others deal with general management issues. Finally, they are at different levels of detail, ranging from high-level business cycles down to complex flow diagrams. They function as analysis and communication devices. They represent the shared or "tribal" knowledge of the organization. They can help transform the management culture to be more analytic.

Consider the complexity of a single business process: dozens of employees, dozens of skill sets, hundreds of data flows, hundreds of steps and tasks, dozens of rooms, hundreds of items of equipment, many policies and procedures, several levels of management, several different departments. Such complexity is difficult to manage without blueprints.

A full-blown planning methodology would provide several volumes of sample outputs. The present book can only provide highlights of the architectural components.

Control Architecture

As mentioned previously, the Control Architecture provides the organizational setting that allows alignment of the other three architectures—Business, Data, and Technical. If a hospital's strategic objective (Business Architecture) is to be the fastest responding hospital in its market segment, but its departments do not agree to use a common Email system (Technical Architecture), then the objective will be adversely offected. If a strategic objective is to pursue managed care aggressively, but systems are not integrated to feed a decision support data base (Data Architecture), then achievement of the objective will be endangered.

Policy on Performance Evaluation: "It is the policy of the hospital to evaluate managers based on two major criteria: (1) achievement of departmental objectives; and (2) contribution to the achievement of other departmental (or enterprise) objectives. Departmental objectives include the standard performance measures for revenues and costs, human resources management (turnover, morale surveys), patient satisfaction, and quality indicators. However, departmental objectives also include effective use of information systems. The hospital establishes measures for the use of information systems by department and it monitors them on a regular basis. Objectives for contribution to other departments' plans will be developed during the strategy and budgeting cycle. The manager establishes his/her own departmental objectives, works with other departments on what they need from him, with particular reference to shared business processes. At the time of performance review, the manager will be evaluated based on his/her internal measures, the assessment of other stakeholder departments, and general contribution to the enterprise goals. Shortfalls on internal measures will be overlooked when offset by contributions to other departments and the enterprise as a whole."

Table 8.2 Outputs of the IS Strategy Process

Activity	Output	Comment
Assess technology	Technology assessment	A matrix matching potential technologies to the hospital's business processes. It should specify the developmental stage of the technology, when it will be broadly adopted, and its costs. This data is widely available from industry publications and consultants.
Internal use of technology	Seven S's analysis	The Seven S's should form the conceptual framework. Is there a fit between the information systems and the strategy? The information systems may have a design that segregates Outpatients from Inpatients, and does not accommodate Home Care patients. This conflicts with a strategy to redesign the business process, making the patient the focus.
	Assessment of application portfolio	For each application, the assessment should evaluate the following: age of application, percent of time spent on maintaining it, number of users, fit with architecture, criticality, "value-added" in terms of the value chain; is it used effectively/properly? For each application, determine the users' view of it: usability, availability, response, quality of documentation, quality of support.
	Service level indicators	Comparison of budgets, portfolios, staff distribution: Determine how the hospital's IS budget compares to that of peer/ competitor hospitals. Categories include capital expenditures, operating expenses, and percent of total hospital operating expenses. It can be difficult to make valid comparisons, since many systems expenses are found in the budgets of user departments.
Set goals & strategy	Mission statement	Includes the systems vision.
	Quantified goals	High-level measures for the department as a whole. They might include project completion percentage, turnover rates, overall system availability, etc.
Develop IT strategy • Control architecture	Policies	Policies for acquisition of information systems; who can do it, who relates new systems to the architecture, standards for connectivity, at all seven levels. This also includes policies on data administration, who is the owner of the data, who is the

(Continued)

Table 8.2 *Continued*

Activity	Output	Comment
		custodian, how security is handled, types of training required for information systems.
	Processes	These represent the methodologies for systems selection, problem investigation, strategic planning, revising the architecture and communicating these revisions, establishment and revision of priorities.
	Organizations	The structure of the organizations that carry out the above policies: which organization makes the systems priorities, the architectural decisions; communications with end users; the strategic plan.
• Business architecture	Strategic model of the industry	This is already available from the strategic plan.
	Value chain	Value chain for each major activity, including links to strategy. Consultants can be useful to the hospital. They can provide instruction and guidance as the hospital performs these activities for the first time. In the long run, however, the hospital must internalize this methodology.
	Reengineered value chain	When this is done, it is frequently found that certain policies contradict each other. This is not surprising, since historically each department's goals were inner-directed. The reengineered value chain must include indicators of success as well as a process for measurement and follow-up. Objectives and incentives must be restructured.
	Organizations	This should provide the details of any organizational structures that ensure quality across departments.
	Improvement opportunities	Initially the hospital will not begin to address all the issues, so this model is a combination of the As-Is and the To-Be.
• Data architecture	Data Model	The Data Model needs to be done in a layered fashion. It is impossible to get the Data Model right on the first pass, but even an incomplete data model is a powerful guide to systems development and integration. There are many automated tools that assist with the creation and maintenance of data models.
	Data dictionary	The data dictionary specifies, for each data item, what it means and where it is found. This is the major tool for an information center.

(Continued)

Table 8.2 *Continued*

Activity	Output	Comment
		• Cross-reference between data model and value chains: This provides important insights for determining those points in the value chain where the systems do not add value.
		• Cross-reference between data model and application-specific files.
• Technical architecture	Standards documents	Physical network, routing, end-user sevices. There should be a published listing of standards and their justification. Where possible, these standards should have an end-user version.
	Cross-reference between business process and systems	For each activity in the value chain, have a table listing its impact on strategy, number of systems accessed, and physical characteristics of its tansactions (frequency, volume, targets).
	Network diagrams	There are several levels of network diagrams. They move one from the logical (user and business) view to the physical (technical and physical) view. One needs both an As-Is and a To-Be diagram.
	Migration plans	For any system/application that will be changed, it is the schedule and impact on the value chain.
Develop IT initiatives	Project plans	Some of these will be infrastructure projects; others will be application projects.
Develop departmental plans	Budgets and plans	Initiatives become projects at the departmental level.

The above policy is a radical departure, both in difficulty of administration and in political acceptability. However, it is necessary.

Policy on Architectural Standards: "It is the policy of the hospital to have connectivity standards for information systems. Any information system being evaluated for acquisition will be analyzed to understand the degree to which it needs to be integrated into the hospital's Business and Technical Architecture. The rankings are from *1* (no need—function is inherently stand-alone) to *5* (core business process—integration required). The hospital maintains a standard evaluation checklist to do this. Systems that score *3* or higher must conform to a set of standards, which include electronic mail, terminal type, network operating system, data base, data access, and remote system access. Waivers will be granted to non-conforming systems based on one or more of the following: security, volume of transactions, short-term acute need. Waivers can be granted only by the IT Steering Committee. If a waiver is given, the installation plan for the system must include a plan for bringing the system into conformance with the Technical Architecture IS within two years. Each year that the system is out of conformance, the sponsoring department will have its IT budget reduced by 10 percent of the system's cost."

Policy on Methodology: "It is the policy of the hospital to require that a 'Business Process Redesign Plan' be developed by any department that is proposing to automate a business process. This document will be developed jointly by IS, management engineering, and the end-user department. The end-user manager is responsible for this document, which will specify the structure of the business process, how it interacts with other business processes, its value detractors, and its improvement opportunities. It will include a blueprint for the redesign of the process, as well as a benefits realization plan."

Policy on IS Organizations: "It is the policy of the hospital to have an IS Steering Committee. Its functions are: (1) to review the information systems plan; (2) to prioritize project requests greater than $50,000; (3) to review and approve changes to the Control Architecture; (4) to review waiver requests; and (5) to review the 'Redesign Plan' for each systems project. There are two levels of steering committee. The tactical level is formed by department heads, who have a greater familiarity with operational details. The strategic level is formed by senior executives. The tactical committee will meet monthly. The strategic committee will meet quarterly."

Business Architecture

Develop a vision statement for each major activity in the cycle, as shown in Figure 8.7 (Outpatient Cycle). This is similar to the vision statement developed when a company does a strategic plan, but at a lower level, moving closer to implementation. It is a way to start establishing/validating goals and measures. In a sense, it becomes a high-level design document against which the current environment is compared. The statement below contains the vision for Outpatient Services.

Outpatient Vision: "Outpatient Operations moves *200* patients a day through the clinic, providing *quality* medical services to patients, with *no more than fifteen-minute* waits; and efficient support to physicians, with *no delays* in delivery of medical records and supplies. This is done through the concerted efforts of Scheduling, Registration, Testing, Treatment, Billing, and Pharmacy. Scheduling

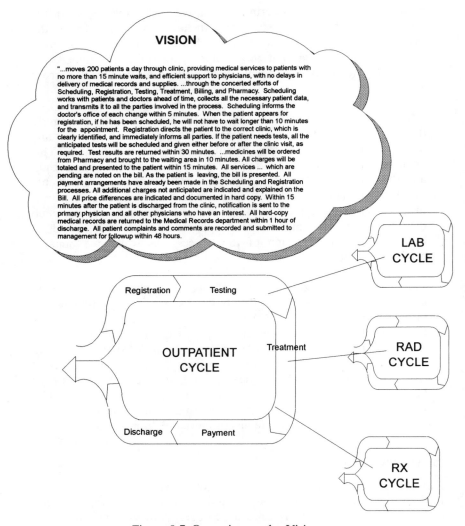

VISION

"...moves 200 patients a day through clinic, providing medical services to patients with no more than 15 minute waits, and efficient support to physicians, with no delays in delivery of medical records and supplies. ...through the concerted efforts of Scheduling, Registration, Testing, Treatment, Billing, and Pharmacy. Scheduling works with patients and doctors ahead of time, collects all the necessary patient data, and transmits it to all the parties involved in the process. Scheduling informs the doctor's office of each change within 5 minutes. When the patient appears for registration, if he has been scheduled, he will not have to wait longer than 10 minutes for the appointment. Registration directs the patient to the correct clinic, which is clearly identified, and immediately informs all parties. If the patient needs tests, all the anticipated tests will be scheduled and given either before or after the clinic visit, as required.   Test results are returned within 30 minutes. ...medicines will be ordered from Pharmacy and brought to the waiting area in 10 minutes. All charges will be totaled and presented to the patient within 15 minutes. All services ... which are pending are noted on the bill. As the patient is leaving, the bill is presented. All payment arrangements have already been made in the Scheduling and Registration processes. All additional charges not anticipated are indicated and explained on the Bill. All price differences are indicated and documented in hard copy. Within 15 minutes after the patient is discharged from the clinic, notification is sent to the primary physician and all other physicians who have an interest. All hard-copy medical records are returned to the Medical Records department within 1 hour of discharge. All patient complaints and comments are recorded and submitted to management for followup within 48 hours.

Registration   Testing

LAB CYCLE

OUTPATIENT CYCLE   Treatment   RAD CYCLE

Discharge   Payment

RX CYCLE

Figure 8.7 Outpatient cycle: Vision.

works with patients and doctors *ahead of time*, collects *all* the necessary patient data, and transmits it to *all* the parties involved in the process. Scheduling informs the doctor's office of each change *within five minutes*. When the patient appears for registration, if he has been scheduled, he will not have to wait *longer than ten minutes* for the appointment. Registration directs the patient to the correct clinic, which is *clearly* identified, and *immediately* informs *all* parties.

If the patient needs tests, *all* the anticipated tests will be scheduled and given either before or after the clinic visit, as required. Test results are returned *within thirty minutes*. After treatment is finished any medicines will be ordered from Pharmacy and brought to the waiting area *in ten minutes*. All charges will be totaled and presented to the patient *within fifteen minutes*. *All* services, such as certain lab results, which are pending, are noted on the bill. As the patient is leaving, the bill is presented. *All* payment arrangements have already been made in the Scheduling and Registration processes. *All* additional charges not anticipated are indicated and explained on the bill. *All* price differences are indicated and documented in hard copy. *Within fifteen minutes* after the patient is discharged from the clinic, notification is sent to the primary physician and *all other* physicians who have an interest. *All* hard-copy medical records are returned to the Medical Records department *within one hour* of discharge. *All* patient complaints and comments are recorded and submitted to management for followup *within forty-eight hours*.

This approach helps all managers and employees see the "big picture." It also helps them refine and formulate the measures at each level of their value chains.

Data Architecture

Much of the analysis done in Chapter 5 would be found in the Data Architecture. In actuality, the Data Model functions very much like the vision statement developed above for the Business Architecture. Its Business Statements and Implications provide a further way to link the non-technical side of the Data Architecture with its more technical, lower level components. Another critical component is the Data Dictionary, which contains definitions for all the entities, attributes, and relationships; the end-user views of the data; and the physical systems in which the entity resides. Table 8.3 presents a sample of this. This mapping is shown graphically in Figure 5.31.

Table 8.3 Data Dictionary Sample

Names employed by end users	Logical entity	Names employed by physical systems
	Account	
Business office		Reg/Billing System
Account number		ACCT_NO in STAY_REC
Registration number		
Billing number		
Laboratory		Lab System
Account number		ACCT_NUM in ACCT_REC
Charge number		

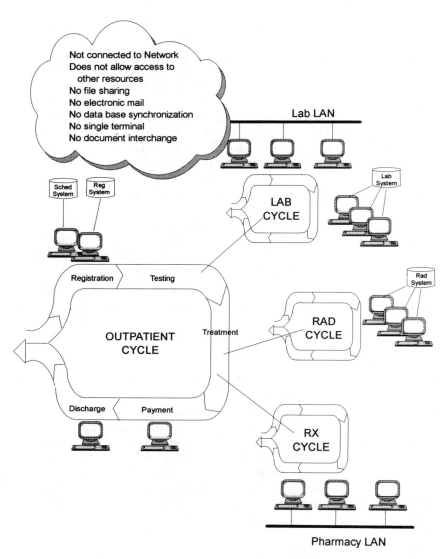

Figure 8.8 Outpatient cycle: As-Is Technical Architecture.

Technical Architecture

The Technical Architecture can be divided into an As-Is model (Figure 8.8) and a To-Be model (Figure 8.9). A technical vision underlies this To-Be model.

Technical Vision: "The hospital's business process are supported by information systems that allow a single terminal to access all the information resources of the hospital, like a large utility. The systems are kept synchronized by real-time exchange of data. While performing his or her function, any hospital employee can alert all other employees by electronic mail. If the employee is doing analysis, s/he can access all other data bases through a common query tool."

From Figure 8.8 one can see the following: The hospital has stand-alone, host-based information systems with direct attachment of dumb

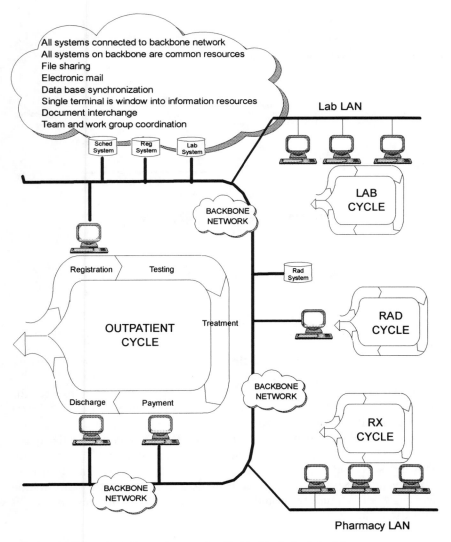

Figure 8.9 Outpatient cycle: To-Be Technical Architecture.

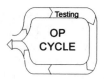

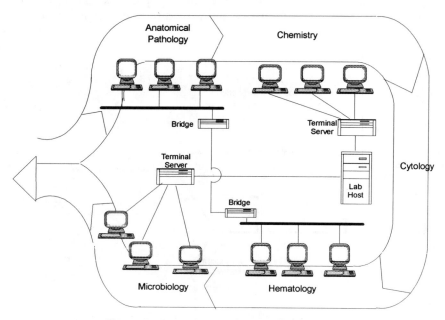

Figure 8.10 Details of As-Is lab architecture.

terminals; there are some stand-alone PCs; the Lab has a Novell network in addition to its Lab host. After this, we could go on to specify how the networks are segmented; where the bridges, routers, and hubs are; the topology for each building; and the design of the wiring closets. A lower level of detail is shown in Figure 8.10.

The same thing will be done for the To-Be Architecture. Subsequent models will take the new logical view and gradually turn it into diagrams showing such physical detail as wiring closets. This gradual transition from business vision to the technical details provides the information systems staff an uninterrupted "audit trail" linking business processes with the technology.

Summary

Having read this chapter, one might conclude that this methodology is impossible to implement; that it imposes too much of an administrative burden on the hospital. Admittedly, people with the wrong skills and the wrong style could turn it into a bureaucratic nightmare. But this has happened with other methodologies as well. Most of the automated tools are available. Those hospitals that have managed to change their culture to a TQM mentality should find this methodology compatible with their new style and structure. Other hospitals, hopefully, will find much that is valuable in it and adopt whatever components they can.

9
Future Issues for Health Care Systems Architecture

This book was written during 1991 and 1992. Great change had already occurred in the health care industry during the 1980s, and even greater change was anticipated for the 1990s. This change will occur along three major dimensions: environment (including economics, demographics, politics, and public opinion), technology, and health care industry structure (including business processes). Both environment and technology will drive changes in industry structure. Many of these factors are inexorable (demographics, global economics), and no amount of hospital preparation will avert them. The challenge for a hospital is to discern the structural changes in broad outline so that it can take advantage of them (or minimize their impact).

Hospitals that plan for change will be more adaptable, even if the predicted changes do not materialize in all their anticipated details. There are certain steps that a hospital can take to become more adaptive: flatten its structure; tighten its control loops; and integrate its data bases. The generic skills acquired from establishing an ongoing TQM/reengineering strategy predispose a hospital to be adaptive. The same can be said for the skills acquired by the "architecting" of information systems.

Health Care Industry Trends

The paradigm of eligibility/coverage/payer/provider/distribution channel can be projected into the future in many different ways, depending on one's political and economic biases. Some experts predict that there will be government-sponsored national health care for all members of the population. Others predict that the government will broaden its eligibility for Medicaid. Still others predict that there will be new entities that arise to provide health care. Regardless of the political solution, several broad structural changes will occur (see Figure 9.1), with universal implications for organizations and their information systems:

- The payers will become more concentrated.
- The providers will become more concentrated.
- There will be new channels of distribution.
- The direct consumer of health care will achieve more leverage over suppliers.
- There will be case management, with emphasis on the total patient.
- Business processes will be redesigned.

Consolidation of Payers

The number of individual payers will shrink, and the size of the remaining payers will grow proportionately. This consolidation of payers will increase their ability to control the prices that they must pay to providers, whether through group rates, managed care, or by dictating specific clinical protocols. Hospitals, through their own initiative and encouraged by government and payers, will streamline administration and billing through

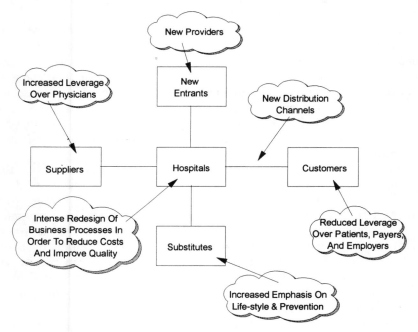

Figure 9.1 Broad structural changes in health care.

standard paperwork and Electronic Data Interchange. Smaller insurers will not be able to institute EDI. There will be increasing social and legislative pressure for insurers to do "community rating" rather than "experience rating," and this will further contribute to consolidation. Government-imposed limits to reimbursement will continue, with private insurers following the same model. Powerful payers will require the reporting of more data by health care providers. This will include cost, satisfaction, and outcome data. Powerful payers will also introduce practice patterns to follow explicit protocols, which will be supported by information systems.

This will cause changes in the business processes of health care providers. It will expand the data model. It will force greater integration across networks, as these "expert" protocols demand real-time data from all ancillary information systems. Data will be requested in greater detail, and with greater frequency. The hospital that does not understand its data, and that does not have a Technical Architecture in place to distribute such data, will fall behind.

Consolidation of Provider Organizations

Economics dictate that hospitals increase their occupancy rate and share expensive medical equipment. Whether forced by the government, encouraged by relaxation of fair-trade practices, or driven by payer leverage, hospital closings and mergers will accelerate. This means that there will be fewer hospitals in a geographical area, and so there will be an increase in smaller entities that can treat patients that do not require an overnight stay. This will also be driven by sociological changes: prevention is beginning to be appreciated more. The patient's condition is a continuum. Organizations that deal with prevention and life-style will have to share data with intervention-oriented organizations.

Consolidation does not refer just to mergers. It also describes the phenomenon of alliances. There is a nascent trend to "mega" medical centers. These "megacenters" are tertiary-care centers that provide a full range of services. As payers consolidate, they will look for economies of scale and higher quality by referring classes of patients (cardiac, transplant, etc.) to a national or regional megacenter. The "centers of excellence" announced by stand-alone hospitals do not necessarily provide all these services at the same level. Government and payers will not want to see massive duplication of facilities and equipment across the institutions of the megacenter. A megacenter will probably be composed of hospitals that are loosely affiliated through participation in the same medical schools. This would require closer coordination of the organizations, a new data model, and more closely coupled information systems. The business flows will have to be redesigned. The data model will have to accommodate multiple medical records for the same patient, unified through a centerwide medical record number.

A similar situation could arise with the chains. While a hospital in Alabama may not ever share the same patients with a hospital in California, the corporate management must make comparisons about relative quality and cost-effectiveness. If the individual hospitals use different information systems, it becomes critical to have a logical understanding of them (done through Data Architecture).

New Distribution Channels

Health care services will be provided through an increasing variety of distribution channels. The microminiaturization of technology, with increasing use of noninvasive procedures, is permitting more work to be done outside of the traditional hospital setting. This is being encouraged by the payers.

Home-based care for the aged will become more frequent. Thanks to high-speed digital networks extending into the home, each bedside could have a physiological data monitor and a computer, connecting the patient with physician, hospital, and ambulance service.

Remote diagnostics, using high-definition television, will extend diagnostic services to new geographical markets. This will reinforce the position of certain medical centers as "megacenters" of excellence.

Traditionally, the design of information systems has been biased toward intervention. Renewed emphasis on prevention will cause organizations to build "health bases"—data bases of the activities of individuals, which will be accessed by hospitals when the person is admitted. This will be relatively "low tech," consisting of data bases and telecommunication links. Individuals will have a terminal at home, and they will enter their daily statistics, which will be forwarded to a larger data base. This larger system will analyze the patient's data, comparing it with peer groups.

All these trends have two major systems implications: connectivity and data interchange, which have been discussed previously. Provider organizations must be in control of their data models to do this.

Greater Attention Paid to Individual Cases

There is a growing interest in correlation of cost, outcomes, and satisfaction at the case level. This is connected with the need to push responsibility for health care consumption to the lowest possible level. All reform parties, no matter what their orientation, agree that there is little or no accountability for the individual's use of health care. The factors that influence this will be studied very intensely. This will require enormous amounts of data collection, connectivity among systems, and expert systems to detect patterns. Large insurers and employers are banding together to develop data bases that will analyze which providers are the most effective along the dimensions of outcomes, service, and cost.

This trend to view the case as a whole is paralleled by a trend to view the patient as a whole. This gives rise to the notion of the "health care cycle." Whereas hospitals have traditionally concentrated on intervention, they will start to deal with a continuum consisting of daily life, checkups, escalation to OP services, escalation to IP services, return to daily life. This, of course, agrees with and reinforces the trend to managed care. The implications for information systems are enormous.

Business Process Redesign

Driven by stronger payers, government, and more informed patients, hospitals will begin to do things differently. This can be seen in out-sourcing, flattening, benchmarking, and reengineering.

Other Issues

Even if health care is nationalized, it will not eliminate private health care, and the related assembly of insurers, providers, and payers. Without implying any value judgment, there will continue to be a "two-tier" delivery system—government versus private. Each of these systems will have its own inherent dynamic. With nationalized health care, probably 70 percent of patients will be covered by the national program, while the remaining 30 percent will choose private health care. As hospitals seek to differentiate themselves from the national system, and from each other, the information systems will diverge. Cost accounting, regulatory reporting, billing, reservations, will all be different. It might prove too difficult for a single type of information system to handle both private health care and national health care. These trends are summarized in Table 9.1.

Technology Trends

Not only environmental change drives industry structure. Technology can also be used to shape the competitive framework of an industry. Advances in information technology allow the innovative hospital to dramatically alter and improve its value chain, which may cause the rules of competition to change, to the hospital's advantage.

Table 9.1 Industry Trends and Their Impact on Strategy

Environmental trend	Structural trends in health care industry	Impact on systems strategy and architecture
Aging population Uninsured population Prevention and life-style Budget deficits Economics, U.S. competitiveness Health care reform Better-informed consumers Technology Growing cost of health care	Consolidation of payers	As payers become more powerful, they will require that hospitals report more data on outcomes, service, and costs. This will dictate electronic links and comparability of data bases. It will also influence practice patterns, which will be taught and enforced with the support of computers. Some hospitals may build a whole strategy around linkages to payers, to turn this payer leverage to their advantage. These hospitals will develop explicit strategies leaders in quality, with every information system designed to enforce, measure, and disseminate quality indicators. These data bases then provide the opportunity to develop value-added services.
	Consolidation of providers	Hospitals will consolidate through mergers, chains, and other innovative affiliations. In the latter case, some hospitals will design their systems to be "interhospital" information systems, allowing maximum affiliation and thus increasing their access to patients and payers. They will have a common backbone network and data interchange to facilitate affiliation.
	New distribution channels	Some hospitals will make it an explicit strategy to maximize distribution channels through electronic linkages and shared data bases. As patients pass through the various phases of the patient cycle (ER → IP → Home Care → OP), they will be able to participate. This will also help in a consolidation strategy, and in a linkage strategy with payers. Payers are demanding a consolidated view for purposes of UR; clinicians will demand the same view, for protocol definition.
	Business process redesign	Some hospitals will make TQM their fundamental strategy, facilitated by the new technologies, which allow dramatic redesign of stand-alone business processes. This will require electronically enforced protocols and real-time systems. There will be electronic linkages among all the institutions that touch the patient's health care cycle. There will be common, or at least comparable, data bases.

Since data is such an integrative factor, it is convenient to classify technology advances in the following way: how they permit data input and output; how they permit data transmission; how they permit data manipulation.

Data Input and Output

Voice Recognition: The ability of a computer to understand human speech. This allows care givers to "talk" their data into the computer, freeing up their hands for patient care and other value-added activities.

Speech Synthesis: The ability of a computer to reproduce human speech. This creates a "talking data base," which can free up the eyes of the care givers.

Miniaturized CRTs: Small display (2 inches diagonally) worn to the side of the eyes, freeing up the eyes of the care giver to concentrate on the patient and eliminate the need to walk away from the patient to refer to documentation.

Hand-held Computers: The size and weight of a small cordless phone. The location of the patient no longer interferes with information capture and retrieval. It goes everywhere with the care giver. The term being used is "Personal Data Assistant (PDA)."

Windows: A standard for the presentation of data to end users. This allows care givers to use multiple systems in the performance of their job, without being distracted by the different appearances of these systems.

Wands and Scanners: Make data capture much less intrusive, and much more accurate.

Sensors: Devices to record changes in a wide variety of phenomena: location, heat, light, body chemistry, and so on. This allows the immediate and accurate capture of a wider variety of data than could ever be done manually. It frees up care givers and also does things they could never do.

Data Transmission

Wireless Networks: Networks that rely on radio waves or infrared waves as the transmission medium. The location of the patient no longer prevents information retrieval. All members of the care-giving team can collaborate through a PDA, and not just beepers.

Digital Public Networks: Traditional telephone networks transmit data using the techniques for voice transmission. They are being revamped to carry high-speed digital transmissions. This means patient homes and other locations can be linked to the care givers.

Data Storage and Organization

Multimedia Data bases: Data bases that accommodate a wide variety of
data types. This allows creation of an "all-electronic" medical record
containing wave forms, images, moving images, voice, handwriting,
and traditional data. Care givers and others can focus on the data,
rather than on the processes required to obtain it.

Knowledge bases: Specialized data bases that encapsulate the knowledge
of clinical experts. They will be available on a network. This facilitates
clinical practice and medical education. It also helps to make standards
of care more uniform.

Data Classification Systems: Methods for unifying the existing systems
for classifying medical data. The Unified Medical Language System
(UMLS) is a superset of CPT and ICD codes. This allows care givers to
focus on the patient.[1]

Data Exchange Standards: HL7 and MEDIX allow systems to be synchronized. This permits greater focus on the data than on the process
to obtain it.

Data Processing and Manipulation

Programming Languages: New languages, more suited for the manipulation of objects, which is required by expert systems and multimedia.

Data Management: Tools to manage the interconnection of diverse data
sources. This includes automated tools to produce and manage
models that underlie the Data Architecture. By 1995–1996 there will
be less discussion of the Layers 1–6 and a commensurately greater
need to deal with the application layer.

Computer-aided Design: Tools to manage the redesign of the business
processes, using computer-aided design (CAD) techniques, as well as
modeling and simulation. Other sets of tools can be used in modeling
patient physiology and simulating clinical procedures.

Application Types

These basic technologies can be combined into software applications,
the tools for supporting patient care. For example, one might combine

---

[1] For an overview of the UMLS, see Donald A.B. Lindberg and Betsy L. Humphreys, "The
UMLS Knowledge Sources: Tools for Building a Better User Interface," *Proceedings of the
Fourteenth Annual Symposium on Computer Applications in Medical Care* (IEEE Computer
Society Press, 1990), pp. 121–125.

networking, optical disks, scanners, and special data base software into a system that provided an electronic chart. In all of this, it is important to remember that these technologies exist only to support the value chain, freeing up humans to do what they do best—diagnosing, treating, comforting, and research.

Niche Systems: Eventually, every function in a hospital will be supported by a "niche" information system. These will all have to be connected.

Groupware: Most software, even though it is used by multiple people, has been developed for stand-alone activity. The software is not aware of the bigger business process in which the user is involved. A new generation of software, called Groupware, knows about the business process (it could be a clinical process as well), and the role that each person (or job class) plays in that business process. Business events trigger other business events. This software can dramatically change the quality of business processes because it prevents data from being lost by informing all concerned parties about the status of the overall process.

Expert Systems: will help many diffferent groups, from clinicians to programmers and IS support staff. Groupware is an expert system since it embodies the knowledge of the business process that a seasoned professional has.

Client-Server: This is technology that distributes application functionality over multiple devices on network. The user's workstation does the data formatting and local processing; a server (or servers) on the network does data management. For example, a legacy application that runs on a mainframe is rewritten to use a powerful DBMS server on a network and the local processing power of the users' PCs. The irony is that, by breaking an application up, one achieves greater integration. The applicability for creating linkages among value chains is obvious.

Virtual Reality: Computers that allow simulation through more than visual feedback. The ultimate in modeling and instruction.

Common Threads

There are several common threads that recur throughout the above-mentioned technology trends. These threads include: Integration, Expert Systems, Ubiquitous Computing, and Data Management.

Integration

Integration is the biggest "megatrend" of hospital information systems. Combining networking, data base management systems, data standards such as HL7 and SQL, as well as new analysis and design methodologies, systems integration enables the integration of the enterprise. As a result, departmental boundaries that impede communication and service will fall, control of business processes will increase, and more enterprise assets will become available to the individual processes.

Standards for Electronic Data Interchange (EDI) will continue to grow. HL7 and MEDIX will be merged. There is increasing interest in merging multiple standards into a single metastandard. Another standard is the MIB (Medical Information Bus). Another aspect of data exchange is SQL (structured query language).

The boundaries between technologies are becoming blurred. Previously, one could expect to find both a physiological data monitor and a CRT in the ICU. Now, these technologies are merging. Physiological data monitors can now transmit waveform data over Ethernet networks, and the same device can be used for both physiological data display and clinical data management. Previously, there had been a strong distinction between accounting data, clinical data, and physiological data. Decision support systems can now integrate the accounting and clinical data. Systems now exist that take snapshots of physiological data and store them in an integrated patient data base.

There is also a blurring of system and enterprise boundaries, not just departmental boundaries. As systems boundaries are redefined, enterprise boundaries are redefined. Hospital information systems increasingly will be linked with the information systems of other organizations, creating interorganizational systems. Such systems can go beyond simple EDI, where one company's system sends a transaction to another company's system, and the latter is free to accept or reject the transaction. Some interorganizational systems allow an "external" organization to use "internal" resources such as entering transactions or browsing the data base. Some interorganizational systems have existed for years. Materials Management is exemplified by the Baxter ASAP system. Hospitals provide physician access to their HIS. Hospitals have connections to external data bases like Medline. In addition, many hospitals have electronic data exchange with payers. Interorganizational systems will be extended to payers and employers, so that they may inspect service, quality, utilization, and cost data. This will also be done with the government. Exchange of patient data will take place more frequently, as hospitals share services in an effort to achieve economies of scale: for example, remote monitoring of high-risk newborns by a pediatric hospital. As data sharing and data exchange increase, additional standards will have to be created for the new transactions.

Interorganizational systems have great implications for both sides, but particularly for the "reacting" organization. Typically, there is an initiator and a reactor. Ideally, such a system should result from a conscious partnership, but frequently the strategy is developed by one organization, which proposes this system to another organization. The proposing organization has thought through the strategic implications and then designed an organization to do it, and finally has designed an information system to do it. This is a top-down approach, as it should be. The reacting organization, however, is likely to take a bottom-up approach, installing the system first, then realizing the organizational implications, and finally realizing the strategic implications. When the reacting organization finally gets to the strategic implications, it may regret not having thought them through at the start of the process. This is illustrated in Figure 9.2.

There is a consolidation of data modalities. Data bases, which formerly housed only text and numeric data fields, can now accommodate voice, handwriting, unstructured text, still pictures, and cinematic images. The data may actually be stored in different physical file structures, but "front-end" software will allow the user to retrieve and manipulate the data as though they were in a single data base. Their physical location can no longer obstruct the business process. All the data will be brought together at a single workstation using a windowed, graphic approach.

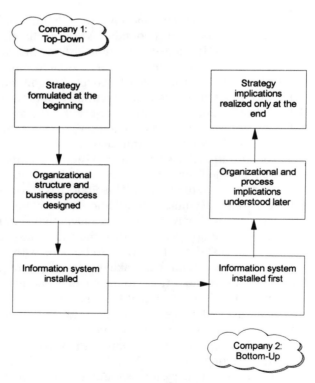

Figure 9.2 Interorganizational system: initiator and reactor.

More and more levels of tools will help the user manage the data. This has major impact on application programs. They will have to be rewritten to take advantage of this. A new generation of design techniques will require object-oriented approaches.

This change will cause the redesign of many business processes, including Medical Records, physician dictation and chart completion, order writing, and so on. For example, the physician no longer must walk down to Radiology to review X-rays; the complete chart will be available to multiple people at the same time—an improvement for teaching hospitals and hospitals that have large, complex outpatient operations. The design of application data bases will have to handle this.

Technology integration has enormous implications for all of the Architectures. The Business Architecture will have to be redesigned to make the best use of it. The Data Architecture will have to change, reflecting different types of enterprises and policies. Most importantly, the Control Architecture will have to change in many respects: organizational rewards, planning, measurement, prioritization, communication formats, team and department structures. The Control Architecture will be the most difficult to resolve.

Dependence on Expert Systems

Expert systems will be embedded in *all* existing application modules, and all new health care information systems will be developed using expert systems technology. It will be used to support activities such as Case Management, Audit, Diagnosis, and Order Entry. This will have profound implications on all aspects of architecture. Activities will be redesigned; networks will have to accommodate the extra data.

Expert systems will really blossom as hospitals and insurers work together to develop protocols for consistency of practice. Vendors will embed expert systems in their modules, or third-party vendors will create "knowledge nodes" on the network, which may be accessed by multiple systems. These third-party knowledge nodes, however, will not be feasible until the industry develops a more detailed clinical data model, which would specify what data elements should be included in a given module, such as Nursing Assessment.

The movement to expert systems is reinforced by trends in data exchange, object-oriented design and development, networking, data capture. HL7/MEDIX types of transactions will be broadcast over the network. In addition to being received by the traditional ancillary systems, they will also be received by "knowledge nodes" which reside on the network. (See Figure 9.3.) These nodes will have expert knowledge of the clinical process and the administrative process; they will have access to all data bases; and, as they are informed of events, they will send out alarms,

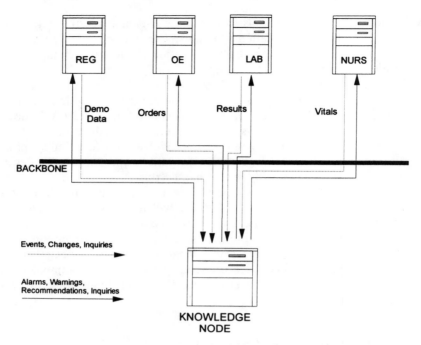

Figure 9.3 Knowledge node on network.

warnings, recommendations, and inquiries to all concerned staff and machines.

This has many different implications.

1. There will be greater demand for real-time fault-tolerant systems. The knowledge nodes cannot be used without constant updates of patient condition. Once human knowledge is embedded in the system and the system becomes the "normal" business process, while humans are the "backup," one cannot tolerate system outages.

2. There will be great demand for "knowledge engineers" rather than programmers, and great demand for new skills and education levels. The Data Architecture will be changed to reflect this new data-driven knowledge in the expert systems.

3. The Business Architecture will change, as jobs and skills, as well as the business processes, are redefined. The embedding of microprocessors in equipment, and the building and the ability to send it in real-time to devices that have human expertise, will cause a drastic redefinition of the control cycles within business processes.

4. The Control Architecture issues will be formidable. A major issue in expert systems is the need to make their knowledge bases accessible and

understandable to the staff who use and maintain them. Many legal questions must be resolved. How are organizations to be structured? How should new systems be developed when there is the possibility to tie them to expert data bases? How should accountabilities be redefined in light of a radically changed control cycle? The difficulties multiply if these expert systems are also interorganizational systems.

Expert systems can help more than medical professionals. "CASE" refers to "computer aided software engineering." This is a special use of expert systems to support the design, development, and maintenance of information systems. The prevailing wisdom dictates that individual hospitals should not attempt to develop large, transaction-oriented applications such as Patient Registration and Order Communications. Few organizations can stand the cost—as much as 100 man-years per module. Few organizations have the resources, technical skills, and methodological sophistication to do this. The problem is that an off-the-shelf product provides generic functionality, perhaps as much as 80 percent of the total required functionality. The lesson: No packaged software will provide competitive advantage to the hospital. However, that unmet 20 percent has the potential to provide sustainable competitive advantage to the hospital, if they can develop it at reasonable cost. This may be changed by CASE technology, whereby a hospital can develop an application that provides a perfect match to its business strategy and processes. What really gives sustainable competitive advantage is an organization (enabled through the appropriate Control Architecture) that can use these CASE tools.

Ubiquitous Computing

Due to microminiaturization, computers will be embedded in every activity and every piece of equipment. Therefore, any activity in the value chain is subject to redesign. Processes can be redesigned to more directly serve their primary goal (patient care, patient service); the current design of many processes reflects the fact that data is not available, is incompatible, or has to be entered and retrieved manually. As mentioned previously, control loops can be redesigned to allow humans to do what they do best—make judgments, care for other humans—while leaving data capture, measurement, storage, and communication to the microprocessors. The fundamental challenge is to change the Control Architecture (culture, reward system, accountabilities, etc.) to allow this redesign.

Data Management

There are many excellent tools for data capture and manipulation, but most are limited in scope—limited in the number of data bases that they recognize, the number of networks over which they run, and so forth.

Table 9.2 Technology Trends and Their Impact on Structural Trends

Technology trend	Structural trends in health care industry	Use of technology to respond to structural trends
Data capture Networking Data bases Expert systems Standards Groupware Integration	Consolidation of payers	As payers (both government and private insurance) become more powerful, hospitals will have to provide greater added value beyond medical services, which will become somewhat more commoditized by standardization forced by the payers. Some hospitals will try to become value-added partners. They will use networking and data bases to redesign their business process (products) for efficiency and quality. They will invest in data capture and networking to measure their quality and share it with the payers. They will also invest in expert systems to establish the clinical protocols that payers will demand. They will do this in real time, and this will be a major value for the payers, as they attempt to do case management.
	Consolidation of providers	Mega medical centers will construct a backbone network to share data about common patients. They will share patients because payers will constrain their ability to acquire expensive duplicate equipment. This backbone will carry all data types: pictures, vital signs, administrative data, etc. As a patient passes through the medical center, all the "stakeholder" hospitals will be informed of his status through EDI. Using wide-area networking, the mega medical center will build a "hub and spoke" arrangement with feeder hospitals in a wide geographical area. At a level below the acuity of the mega medical center, chains will grow. Some chains will adopt a strategy of value-added, providing maximum data to insurers and payers, using networks, data capture technology, and data bases.
	New distribution channels	Some hospitals will adopt a strategy of dealing with the *total patient*, across all phases of the health care cycle: wellness, checkups, outpatient treatment, inpatient treatment, skilled nursing, home health care, and back to wellness. They will use networking and data bases to integrate all modes of service delivery and provide this data to insurers and payers. Expert systems will be used to assist in the delivery of care.

(*Continued*)

Table 9.2 *Continued*

Technology trend	Structural trends in health care industry	Use of technology to respond to structural trends
	Business process redesign	Many hospitals will use networking to restructure the business processes that underlie their medical services. Some may go to "just-in-time" inventory methods. They will outsource non-core functions. One candidate is the operation of data centers and networking. As networks become more standardized, and as Level-7 standards connect more and more applications, hospitals can outsource these activities and concentrate on developing high-impact information systems to support key activities.

Probably the best way to ensure an integrative mapping from the Data Model to individual systems is through a "heterogeneous Distributed Data base Management System" that coordinates all other data management activities of the individual systems. This, in a sense, is another knowledge node on the network. It represents the knowledge of the human "data architect." It is a system that has a catalog of all the data that needs to be integrated, where it resides, and how to access it. This is probably a better way to achieve synchronization than the current method of each system sending its own HL7 transactions across a network. Research to achieve this goal is being done by many vendors. This will provide the "logical glue" that will facilitate the integrative power of the previously-mentioned technologies. Once again, the effective use of such data base management systems will require changes to the Control Architecture. Who is responsible for defining the data model, for maintaining it, for enforcing it? How can departments share responsibility for the integrity of an entity's attributes? Who is responsible for enforcing the Data Architecture when systems are developed? How does the reward system reinforce good corporate citizenship with regard to data?

Impact on Hospital Value Chains

Hospitals can take advantage of these technology trends, to use them as catalysts in changing their business processes to respond strategically to the structural changes in the industry. These approaches are summarized in Table 9.2.

10
Mock Strategic Plan

This chapter tries to synthesize the book's material by simulating the information systems strategic plan for a fictitious hospital. Tri-City Children's Hospital (TCH) is a 350-bed children's hospital located in a major urban area. It is part of a large medical center and is affiliated with a medical school. For most of its existence, TCH was actually part of an adult critical-care hospital. Several years ago, it was decided that TCH should be set up as an independent entity, with its own separate employees, departments, buildings, and systems. For the past six years TCH has had an implicit strategy of separation and stabilization. It had to construct new buildings, recruit staff, acquire equipment and technology, and set up business policies and procedures. Now, all that has been completed, and TCH has started to develop a 5-year plan. The 1990s will be a time of great change for the United States in general and for hospitals in particular.

In preparation for the next 5–10 years, TCH has been working with consultants to develop a strategic plan to carry the hospital through the 1990s. While it was never explicitly articulated, TCH has had a de facto plan for the past six years: build the infrastructure of a new hospital. The objectives have all been achieved:

1. Three new buildings have been constructed.

2. Three thousand employees have been hired and trained.

3. An endowment fund has been established, and it is worth $500 million.

4. Operations of twenty-four new departments have been established and stabilized.

5. Medical technology and information technology have been acquired and installed.

6. Clinical excellence has been maintained in the face of this change.

We, the strategic planning team, decided that now that we have built this infrastructure, we need to move into the 1990s and beyond. We asked ourselves who we were and what we want to be. Until now, we have been the dominant children's hospital in our geographical region. We have had a favorable payer mix and good reimbursement rates, little managed care, and a solid endowment. Our employee turnover rates, while fairly high, are no higher than that of our peers. Because of our relative profitability and monopoly position, we have not paid much attention to issues of efficiency and patient satisfaction.

However, we are moving into a period of great instability for health care. The economic, political, and social environment is changing, and will continue to do so. TCH is going to have to adapt to this. A significant factor in this is information technology. This part of the strategic plan focuses on how IS will support our strategic activities.

External Environment

The team looked at the trends in the external environment: politics, demographics, economics, and so on. It found that major structural realignments have been occurring in all these areas. The findings are the following:

1. In every major city, large employers have formed a coalition to give them leverage against hospitals. They are building comprehensive data bases of diagnoses, outcomes, costs, and patient satisfaction. It is a natural step to boycott hospitals that do not conform to the average; conversely, hospitals that are above average will receive more business. This will eventually become a national data base.

2. Large employers are reducing the amount of benefits available to employees in their health care coverage, and are introducing more and more "managed care" features into their packages. "Managed care" is defined to be the following: a data-oriented approach to patient care, which projects demand for services based on the demographics of the patient population and historical trends; which budgets costs based on this projected demand; and which concentrates on the close management of each case to determine the appropriate level of care. This approach requires great understanding of one's costs and patients, as well as systems

to control costs and to manage patients in real time throughout the cycle of pre-sickness, sickness, and post-sickness. Payers are becoming more organized and more consolidated. They will demand more consistent, mutually agreed-upon clinical protocols.

3. Medical centers are getting larger. Employers and insurers are developing agreements with large centers for the centers to become their exclusive providers for many services. Medical technology accounts for about 25 percent of all health care costs. Research has documented that the more frequently a hospital performs a given procedure, the better its outcomes. This is a natural outcome of experience. This will cause some hospitals to divest their technology, when it turns out that employers and insurers divert their patients to facilities with a better record.

4. Hospitals will protest that the data bases are unfair, that their patients are really sicker than average, or that there are some other extenuating circumstances. This will lead to the creation of more sophisticated information systems that will track multiple types of data for each of the major parameters: patient, diagnosis, treatment, cost, and satisfaction.

5. The percentage of gross national product consumed by health care is growing. In 1992 it consumed about 14 percent of GNP; in 1993 it will probably consume 15 percent. The impact of this on the ability of U.S. companies to compete in global markets has been noted. At the same time, indicators for quality of health and quality of life are not improving at the same rate, or at all. This reinforces the trends in cost control and prevention/life-style.

6. It is becoming clearer that intervention, symbolized by technology, is not effective, and that medicine must emphasize prevention and life-style. This attitude is further strengthened by the situations regarding prenatal care, child care, and immunizations.

7. The number of uninsured people is growing, and thus the number of uninsured children. This damages national morale. More specifically, it causes people to use the Emergency Room for primary care. It also means that people present themselves in a much more critical condition than they would if they had access to affordable primary care. This means that TCH and other hospitals have to cost-shift; that is, make up the shortfall by overcharging other customers. This will not be continued because, as the employers drive the hospitals to perform managed care, the costs will be identified and hospitals will not be able to cost-shift.

8. The number of family-oriented organizations is growing. This indicates a change in attitudes toward children. This, combined with emphasis on prevention, can either help or hurt TCH, depending on how it approaches the prevention issue.

9. For Medicare patients, the government has started to restructure its reimbursement rates, favoring primary care and prevention, while constraining specialties such as surgery and high-tech procedures (that is, the

subspecialties). This will probably be copied by the major insurers and employers.

10. Health care will be reformed, in one way or another. During 1992–1993, Congress had before itself over thirty proposals for the reform of health care delivery and financing. They included comprehensive restructuring proposals, such as national health care, to more "tinkering" proposals such as tort reform. President Clinton has made health care reform his first priority, and he is inclined to create greater government involvement. However, regardless of the form taken by the ultimate political solution, the health care system of the future will surely have the following general characteristics: emphasis on managed care; consolidation of services into regional/national centers; prevention; greater government regulation; and documentation of the balance among cost, quality, satisfaction, and severity.

11. Technology is becoming microminiaturized and virtual. By virtual, we mean that a physician can deliver services as though he were actually there. Examples of this are HDTV (high-definition TV).

12. There is an ongoing shortage of technical staff for hospitals. This includes registered nurses, radiology technicians, lab technicians, and so on. Medical students for the past ten years have been going into subspecialties at an increasing rate. General Pediatrics and Primary Care have suffered because of this.

13. While the country is experiencing a "mini baby boom" and children's hospitals have high occupancy rates, the low occupancy rates of other hospitals may lead them to try to "poach" patients from children's hospitals. Obviously, patient age and travel distance will limit the feasibility of poaching as a strategy.

14. The trend to Total Quality Improvement, has begun to spread to health care. This appears to be a serious movement. The implicit foundation of this is that the ultimate strategic advantage is provided by the employees and the organizational structure that empowers them. As the data bases on satisfaction, outcomes, and costs grow, and as the fight to find and retain employees continues, those hospitals that successfully adopt a TQM approach will be winners on several fronts.

15. There are several major trends in information systems: open systems standards and products, data bases, networks, and clinical systems. They provide a powerful catalyst for business process redesign.

Tri-City Children's Hospital Environment

Performance Measures

1. TCH has been profitable. This has allowed us to build the new wings and to acquire the latest in medical equipment and information tech-

nology. The problem is that we do not know how long this is going to last we have been profitable under the *old paradigm*, which is changing.

2. TCH has managed to reduce the turnover rate, and hold it to 20 percent annually. This is fair, but it needs to be improved if we move to a TQM position.

3. Patient demographics have remained relatively stable for the past five years.

4. The mix of payers has started to change. There has been a consistent decline in the number of Blue Cross and other private indemnity-based insurers; the percentage of managed care patients has increased; and the percentage of Medicaid patients has increased. The Medicaid reimbursement ratio is a fragile thing, and any change to it could greatly impact the hospital. There is a limit to the amount of cost-shifting that the hospital can do.

5. We have not been doing a good job in tracking the satisfaction of patient families. One school of thought argues that it is not important to track the satisfaction of Medicaid patients, since they do not pay anyway. On the other hand, the government is becoming very interested in what they think about the hospitals they use.

6. We have not been doing a good job in training. Each year, investment in capital assets is fifty times the amount of money spent on the training of our human assets. However, salaries account for 70 percent of the operating budget.

7. Since this portion of the strategic plan concerns information systems, we have placed their performance evaluation into a separate section.

8. We do not have a strong understanding of our costs, and we do not have a methodology for the costing of our services. Government, employers, and insurers are demanding that costs be correlated with services and outcomes. We cannot do that analysis with any granularity of detail. We do not have a strong understanding of profitability by product line. Some services probably lose money by themselves, but draw patients to the hospital to use other services. However, we cannot prove this.

TCH Information Systems Trends

The state of our information systems is mixed. Most equipment is modern, if not state of the art. We have a backbone network, but we do not take advantage of it to integrate applications and departments. Every major department is automated, but this has been done without a strategic plan and architecture.

The team surveyed the users to learn how they view the state of TCH's information systems. The general pattern is that TCH's information systems have good functionality for the accounting and administrative func-

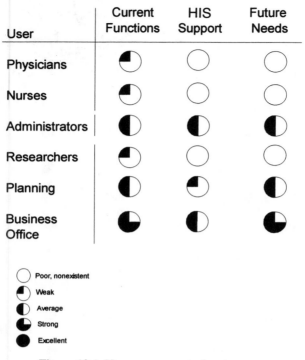

User	Current Functions	HIS Support	Future Needs
Physicians	◕	○	○
Nurses	◕	○	○
Administrators	◑	◑	◑
Researchers	◕	○	○
Planning	◑	◕	◑
Business Office	◕	◑	◕

○ Poor, nonexistent
◔ Weak
◑ Average
◕ Strong
● Excellent

Figure 10.1 User assessment of systems.

tions, but are weak in supporting the clinical side of the hospital, and do not provide any integration. Support for accounting and administration is average, but nonexistent for clinical users. (See Figure 10.1.) This reflects the fact that HIS reports to the chief financial officer (CFO). Probably HIS will need to be reorganized to report to a CIO with a clinical background. The trend to TQM will require leadership that understands the hospital processes.

We also surveyed users and IS staff about each system, and compared this to data concerning our peer children's hospitals. This data supports the first survey. TCH is competitive with its peers regarding accounting, administration, and individual ancillaries. It lags its peers in support of physicians, nurses, researchers, and in integration. See Figure 10.2.

In addition, we examined the IS staff to determine whether it has the skill base required in light of the major trends and TCH strategies. We found them deficient in several major areas (see Figure 10.3).

We also reviewed the existing Control Architecture (although no one calls it by that name). TCH exhibits a strong preference for vertical structures and departmental orientation. This is illustrated in Figure 10.4.

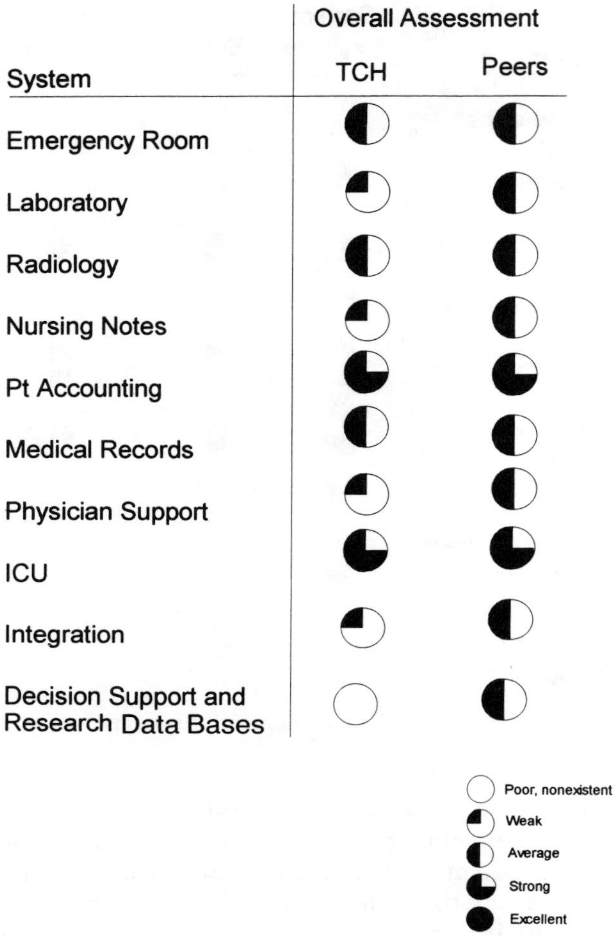

System	Overall Assessment	
	TCH	Peers
Emergency Room	◐	◐
Laboratory	◔	◐
Radiology	◐	◐
Nursing Notes	◔	◐
Pt Accounting	◕	◕
Medical Records	◐	◐
Physician Support	◔	◐
ICU	◕	◕
Integration	◔	◐
Decision Support and Research Data Bases	○	◐

Legend:
○ Poor, nonexistent
◔ Weak
◐ Average
◕ Strong
● Excellent

Figure 10.2 Assessment of TCH vis-à-vis peers.

The result is an Era I mentality within the HIS department and an Era II mentality among the end user departments, preventing the creation of an effective architecture. These issues will have to be addressed, both in HIS and in the general hospital, before any major new strategic initiatives are undertaken.

Strategic Options

The team looked at the feasibility of continuing the past practices; in other words, doing nothing. This was rejected universally. Under the

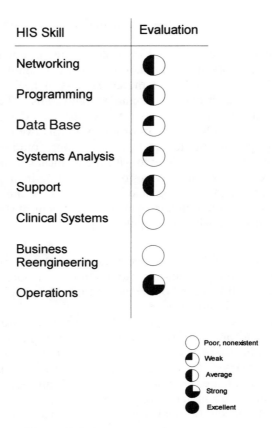

HIS Skill	Evaluation

Figure 10.3 Assessment of HIS skills.

Control Architecture

Component	Centralized	Vertical
Reward System	Y	Y
Organizational Structures	Y	Y
Prioritization System	Y	Y
Standards Setting System	Y	Y
Culture	Y	Y
Planning System	Y	Y

Figure 10.4 Assessment of control architecture.

change scenario, we examined multiple options in our response to managed care, consolidation, human resources, technology, quality, and demographics. It is clear that the consumers of health care are gaining leverage over the providers, including physicians. The hospital should recognize this and move aggressively to adapt to this new environment and turn it to our advantage. In order to do this, we have recommended the following four broad strategic directions, outlined below. These strategies need to be coordinated with the medical side of the house: their ongoing programs for quality control, as well as their plans for product innovation through teaching and research. It is the intention of the hospital to obtain the full participation of the medical staff in the strategic planning process, beginning in 1994.

1. *Managed care*: TCH will integrate principles of managed care into its philosophy and operations. No matter what solution is ultimately developed, it will be based on managed care. Hospitals that do not adapt to this practice will not survive.

2. *Quality*: TCH will integrate TQM principles into its management philosophy and practice. This will impact every one of its business processes. For the past twenty years American industry has been working harder, not smarter. TQM will enable TCH to work smarter, with fewer employees and greater employee retention. Ultimately, TQM will reduce costs and allow us to more effectively measure, document, and communicate our levels of quality to a marketplace that will examine it closely.

3. *Consolidation*: TCH will become a "mega" medical center for pediatric care. There are too many hospitals, with too many unoccupied beds and unused equipment. As payers and employers consolidate, they will seek to gain economies of scale and higher quality by contracting with fewer, but larger, health care entities. This may require building new facilities. It may also require extending our geographical markets and professional relationships with other providers.

4. *Prevention*: TCH will become the leading medical center for treating the "whole" child, by taking a "life cycle" approach to health care, in which prevention and education play a prominent role. This may seem unusual for a tertiary-care institution, but it is simply the extension of TQM principles, which exhort us to look for and solve underlying causes, not symptoms.

In addition to these new strategies, we will maintain existing strategies for areas such as government relations, public relations, and fund-raising.

While developing these broad strategies, the team examined the ways in which information systems could help implement them.

1. *Managed Care*: This is very data intense. Information Technology could help acquire data base systems to track patients by diagnosis, cost, physician, outcome, satisfaction, and severity. IT could also be used to close the operations cycle, providing prospective access to employers, real-time access when a patient is hospitalized (both local and remote), and post-discharge tracking. IT will also be useful in marketing managed care products in terms of projecting profitability and demand, as well as in marketing and negotiating activities.

2. *Total Quality Improvement*: While Total Quality Management will cause the hospital to "reengineer" its business process for the special area of managed care, this strategic direction eventually will cause the hospital to examine every activity and reengineer many of them. Once again, information technology can prove invaluable. One of the assumptions of TQM is that one quantifies and measures as many activities as possible. It also requires that one provides data to employees on the spot, so that they are empowered to make decisions. Finally, as the business processes are redesigned, information systems will have to be acquired to support them, or existing information systems will have to be modified.

3. *Consolidation*: Tri-City Children's will get out in the forefront of consolidation and become a megacenter for pediatric care. This will have enormous implications for all areas of the hospital. Medical staff will have to recruit specialists with an international reputation in order to draw patients from other states and countries. Marketing will have to work with medical staff to help them target large areas of demand. Medical staff will have to improve its research areas to be world class. Registration and medical records will have to deal with patients from other states and countries. Billing will have to deal better with foreign countries, perhaps establishing special relationships with foreign banks. Additional facilities will have to be built to accommodate an increase in the number of patients and the number and frequency of services. An ancillary issue arises: how to house parents of children who come from other states for a stay of several days or longer. Children who are older are more likely to be transported out of state. New legislation allowing parents to take off from work will help. Information systems will provide integration of data bases and a communications network to support the close coordination of the activities of multiple organizations.

4. *Prevention*: Tri-City Children's will alter its philosophy and model of practice to integrate prevention and education into it. Both the public (consumers, employers, insurers) and government are changing their attitudes, and this must be accommodated. It is the right thing to do, plus it will win their favor when they have to make judgments that will affect our hospital. This means that TCH will introduce preventive activities such as education, immunizations, child protection services, and so forth. Once again, information systems will help to integrate the diverse organizations that deal with the different stages of the wellness cycle.

All of this has profound implications for the organization and its information systems. The latter could be used in redesign, marketing data bases, interorganizational connections, and research facilities. The IT vision is that a clinician, using a workstation connected to the TCH backbone network, has windowed access to external facilities, such as Medline; access to all the physical data bases in the hospital; and an electronic medical record. The clinician has query and extract capability from each system and modeling, graphics, and word processing; plus electronic mail to all parties, both in the hospital and outside. Such a scenario, while not sufficient, is certainly necessary to help the hospital attract world-class researchers and diagnosticians.

Information Systems Strategy Options

The team examined which HIS strategies might be employed to achieve the above vision. No matter which approach is taken, the assessment of HIS skills (Figure 10.3) and of the TCH Control Architecture (Figure 10.4) show that investment will have to be made in HIS staff, and staff throughout the hospital will have to be empowered and linked horizontally. The overall approach is the following: (1) Combine process redesign activities with systems development projects; (2) buy third-party packages and focus on their integration; (3) leverage consultant skills, guaranteeing knowledge transfer through contractual stipulation; (4) develop and maintain explicit architectures; (5) be an early adopter of technology, not a leading-edge adopter or a late adopter; (6) invest heavily in the training and empowerment of HIS staff. The rationales and implications behind these HIS strategies are provided below.

Process Redesign: This is one of the fundamental strategies of the hospital, and must be adopted by every department. Historically, TCH has tried to solve business process problems by mechanically automating them, instead of redesigning them and then deciding how to automate them. This has been reinforced by an organizational culture that stressed short-term, reactive activity; lack of HIS methodology; and lack of skills, both in HIS and in end-user departments.

Integrate Third-Party Packages: TCH has consistently chosen to purchase large applications, and will continue to do so, since they are too costly and time-consuming to be developed in-house. However, TCH has never integrated the applications. This will be required by Process Redesign. A major issue for each future system acquisition will be the "integratability" of the package. Obviously, the technology for integration has improved over time, and has not always been available. But even when it has been available, it has not been used. This results from the same problems discussed in Process Redesign: an organizational culture that stressed short-term, reactive activity; lack of HIS methodology; and lack of skills, both in HIS and in end-user departments. TCH will have to develop its integration strategies and provide the tools and skills to its staff, which are currently missing. While self development of applications such as Patient Registration or Medical Records is clearly out of the question, decision-support data bases are candidates for internal development.

Leverage Consultants: Finding and retaining qualified staff will continue to be an issue. Therefore, in large integration and/or application development efforts, consultants will be used to accelerate TCH's ascent of the technical learning curve. Historically, TCH has not made any effort to measure the degree of knowledge transfer resulting from a consulting engagement. All contracts with consultants will be written to ensure measures of knowledge transfer to HIS staff, and payment will be tied to this. A further aspect of this strategy is the need to maintain a "stable" of qualified HIS managers who can manage the consultants. Previous consulting engagements have suffered from a lack of direction and a certain amount of self-serving behavior on the part of the consultants. This can be explained by HIS's failure to manage the consulting effort. The cause of this: top management is reluctant to empower HIS staff. One final aspect of this strategy is the need to train the consultants as well. In order to maximize consultant effectiveness, they will receive a consultant's orientation package to the hospital.

Early Adopter of Technology: TCH has been, and will continue to be, an early adopter of technology. This means that once a technology has been shown to be effective in several hospitals, not necessarily pediatric facilities, TCH will examine it for adoption. It is a leading-edge adopter of medical technology, and this is appropriate, given TCH's standing among pediatric institutions. However, it will not accept the risk and expense of being a leading-edge innovator in information systems. However, TCH must adopt IS technology fairly early in its life cycle, to support its numerous clinical innovations. In the past, TCH has acquired technology fairly early in its life cycle, but has not used it effectively. This weakness will be addressed by the use of consultants.

Invest in HIS Staff: With regard to staffing, the hospital will hire permanent, highly qualified staff to support the systems. The question arises: To what extent can a hospital achieve strategic advantage through the use of information systems technology? There may be a certain advantage to being a "first mover"; however, that requires an even bigger investment in equipment and staff. We will acquire and use technology faster and more adroitly than other children's hospitals. After technology becomes diffused, however, there is no inherent advantage to it. It then becomes the case that the ultimate strategic advantage is in one's *use* of the information systems, and that is a *human resources* issue. TQM will help in this area. This means a big investment in recruiting and retention of HIS staff. We will provide more training than any other children's hospital. We will make a conscious effort to involve HIS staff in hospital operations at least twice a year, for a period of three days each. Skills include communications and presentations, health care industry knowledge, data base, systems analysis and design, expert systems, C++, hypertext systems, networking, instruction. We will also need to recruit a CIO, whose hallmark will be broad experience, good technical background, and outstanding people skills. We will quantify these skills as we do recruiting. Outsourcing has been considered, and has not been excluded. However, it will be done only for those HIS services that are utility-like in nature. This would include data center operations, network management, and Help Desk for generic software tools such as WordPerfect and Lotus. Other value-added activities, such as HIS application support, systems development and process reengineering, and Archtecture are too closely linked to the hospital value chains to be outsourced.

IS Controls

Information Systems will work closely with top management to establish the Control Architecture that will allow the hospital to integrate its systems with its business processes. These controls will include technical standards, organizations, methods, and rewards. They will be outlined initially; then the details will be filled in, over time, as infrastructure projects.

Strategic Initiatives and Departmental Projects

In order to begin implementing the new strategies, individual departments, in collaboration with the strategic planning team, have defined the following multiyear initiatives.

Strategy 1: Managed Care

Initiative: Establish managed care arrangements with two major insurers that have traditionally refused to use TCH services.

Marketing: Will establish a structure for the coordination of managed care products. They will set up a data base for analysis of the profitability of the managed care lines. They will design a program and market it to large insurers and self-insured employers.

Nursing and Physicians: Will examine product lines for feasibility within a managed care approach, and redesign them. They will design new patient flows, protocols for care, team approaches, as well as control and analysis systems.

Finance: Will perform income/expense projections for managed care programs. They will also create pricing structures.

Strategy 2: Total Quality

Initiative: Select two product lines that cut across a representative number of business process and redesign them according to a TQM model. This will have creative overlap with the first initiative. It should be emphasized that "quality" refers primarily to the business process aspects of hospital activities (as discussed in Chapter 4), not to the clinical aspects.

Nursing: Will establish a model and methodology for TQM. This will be done on a pilot basis, with two General Nursing floors participating. Part of the model will address issues of organizational structure and reward and measurement systems.

Business Services: Will do the same as Nursing. The coordinator of the overall initiative will ensure that the methodologies are not contradictory.

Ancillary Departments: All departments whose value chains intersect those of the processes selected for TQM redesign will participate. Like Business Services, they will develop models and methods that complement those developed by Nursing.

Strategy 3: Prevention

Initiative: Define a model for the total wellness of patients and establish close affiliations with organizations that deal with phases other than the tertiary-care phase. Redesign the hospital activities that could support these affiliations. It is difficult for TCH to do this alone, since it receives its patients only by referrals from community physicians and other hospitals. There is a fair amount of risk in this initiative, inasmuch as it requires dealing with governmental agencies driven by political expediency and having no long-range strategy. However, it helps shape public opinion to understand the nature of the hospital's services, and it reinforces the channels of patient supply.

Marketing: Working with clinical staff, will approach other health care organizations about establishing closer affiliation. Part of this activity will be to understand how TCH can have a more favorable impact on that organization's value chain. Marketing will go on to develop materials for public relations and advertising.

Nursing and Physicians: Will develop a model for the total patient, defining explicitly how TCH fits into the model, and how it provides value to other organizations that are concerned with the other phases of the patient's wellness cycle.

Finance: Will perform income/expense projections for these affiliations. They will also create pricing structures.

Strategy 4: Mega Medical Center

Initiative: Develop plans and expand hospital to be positioned as a mega medical center.

Facilities: Will develop a feasibility plan for a new patient-care tower and a facility to house parents from remote cities and states. They will also develop plans for satellite sites.

Marketing and Strategic Planning: Will develop a feasibility plan for building a network of "feeder" hospitals. They will also develop a plan

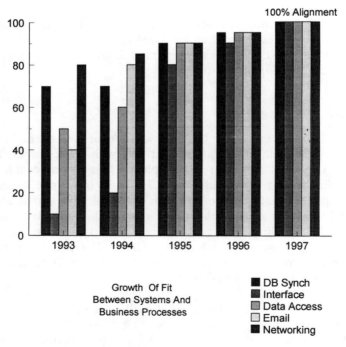

Figure 10.5 Growth of fit between systems and business processes.

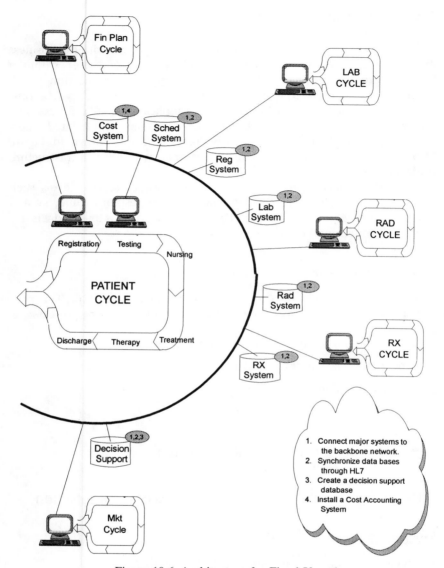

Figure 10.6 Architecture for Fiscal Year 1.

for marketing the expanded facility to employers and insurers on both a national and international basis.

Nursing and Medical Staff: Will develop models for product line placement and patient-care structure in a decentralized environment.

Five-Year Information Systems Plan

This plan is designed to achieve alignment of the systems with the business processes. The word "alignment" means that the end user within a business process sees the following: (1) a network connection to all other resources, (2) a consistent screen that can access all applications, (3) synchronization of all data across applications, (4) access and manipulation of all data, (5) Email, file exchange, and related interaction with all other users. The schedule for this is shown in Figure 10.5. There are many technical details that will form infrastructure projects.

In addition, each year's objectives include target service levels such as system availability, project deadlines, system response time, system integrity, and help desk response. The economic analysis and budgets are being performed by the finance department.

Systems Plan for Fiscal Year 1

Some of the technical details are illustrated in Figure 10.6. The plan represents a balance between applications and infrastructure projects:

1. Connect major systems to the backbone network
2. Synchronize data bases through HL7
3. Create a decision support data base
4. Install a Cost Accounting System
5. Other
   - Maintain existing systems at agreed-upon levels
   - Upgrade Registration computer

The strategic benefits of these projects are explained in Table 10.1.

Systems Plan for Fiscal Year 2

The technical details are summarized in Figure 10.7.

1. Install common electronic mail
2. Add connectivity to local hospitals and physician offices
3. Install a Nursing system
4. Install a Human Resources system

5. Other
   - Install centralized, computerized Help Desk
   - Maintain existing systems at agreed-upon levels

The strategic benefits of these projects are explained in Table 10.2.

Systems Plan for Fiscal Year 3

The technical details are summarized in Figure 10.8.

1. Develop Clinical decision support data base

2. Install common SQL

3. Install electronic links to payers, employers

4. Add standard interface (Windows) for users

5. Other
   - Maintain existing systems at agreed-upon levels
   - Gateways to ICU from clinical DSS

The strategic benefits are summarized in Table 10.3.

Systems Plan for Fiscal Year 4

The technical details are summarized in Figure 10.9.

1. Install quality decision support data base

2. Connect imaging systems

3. Install Prototype of electronic medical record

4. Install networks in new building

5. Other
   - Maintain existing systems at agreed-upon levels
   - Examine feasibility of expert systems

The benefits are summarized in Table 10.4.

Systems Plan for Fiscal Year 5

This will be a year for major architecture review. As more applications are identified in yearly planning during years 2–4 they will be included in Fiscal Year 5.

Table 10.1 Fiscal Year 1 Plan

Goals	Strategy benefits			
	Managed care	Total quality	Consolidation	Prevention
Major systems on backbone	Data access for analysis and reporting of utilization and costs	Allows clinical area to see what the others are doing, can lead to higher quality	Permits connection to other organizations	Everyone involved with the wellness cycle can view patient data
Synchronize data bases	Prerequisite for data access	Required by higher quality	Allows other physicians and providers to have access to unified picture	Patient will be found in various data bases that support different segments of the cycle
Decision support data base	To analyze services by geographical area, which HMOs are we working with	First step to providing a total integrated view of patient and hospital	Can be expanded to include comparative and consolidated data	Can help us understand our client population better, for preparation of educational materials
Cost accounting	Without cost data, managed care is not feasible	Cost is an important factor in the quality equation		

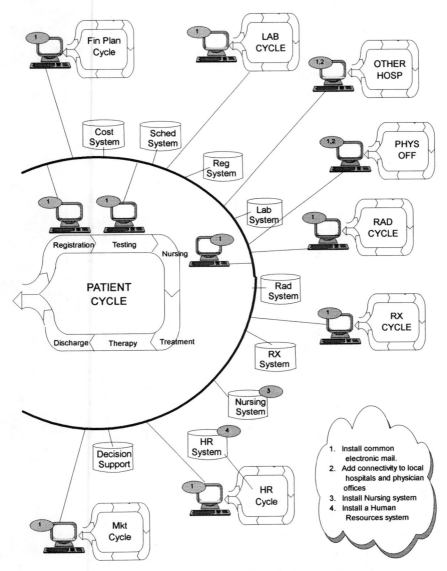

Figure 10.7 Architecture for Fiscal Year 2.

Table 10.2 Fiscal Year 2 Plan

Goals	Strategy benefits			
	Managed care	Total quality	Consolidation	Prevention
Common electronic mail	Communication of trends to payers Infrastructure issue—needed for all process redesign	Broadcast of quality alerts Unifies quality teams Interaction without meetings	Facilitates management communication with other organizations	Distribution of educational materials
Connections to local hospitals and physician offices	Facilitates concurrent case management	Concurrent case management	Increases the referral base for the extended organization	Distribution of educational materials
Nursing system	Better scheduling of resources	Faster and more accurate input of data Data becomes available to all clinicians	Helps to ensure standards of care across multiple organizations	
Human resources system	Helps with productivity measurement	Reduces nursing turnover Tracks skills and training of critical staff	Allocation of skills across the extended organization	

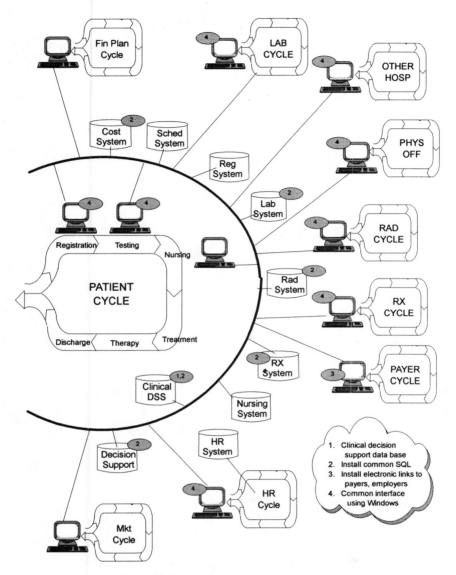

Figure 10.8 Architecture for Fiscal Year 3.

Table 10.3 Fiscal Year 3 Plan

Goals	Strategy benefits			
	Managed care	Total quality	Consolidation	Prevention
Clinical decision support data base	Helps develop clinical protocols Can be combined with other data bases Evaluate staff, outcomes, and resource use	Helps with medical education	Ensures standards for quality across organizations	Can be used to develop educational materials
Common SQL Electronic links to payers and employers	Integrated view of all data about managed care Payers and employers see extra value and proof of our outcomes Faster and more accurate communication	Integrated view of all quality data Reinforce redesign of process to provide value-added to payers (quality data)	Integrated view of all organizations Used by all organizations in the extended enterprise	Used in research on disease patterns
Windows for interface	All information systems for managed care easier to use, more integrated	All information systems for Quality easier to use, more integrated	Integrates the enterprise	Preparation of instructional materials

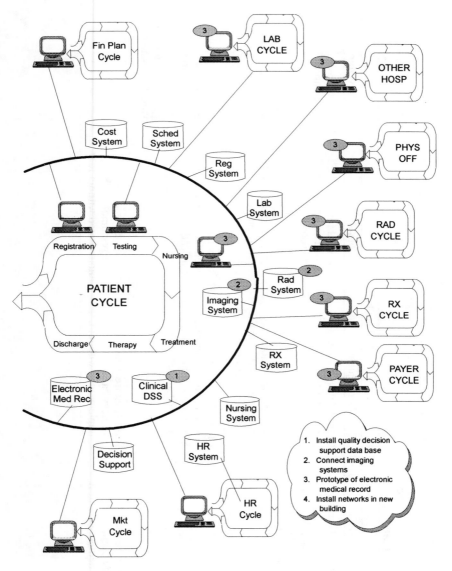

Figure 10.9 Architecture for Fiscal Year 4.

Table 10.4 Fiscal Year 4 Plan

Goals	Strategy benefits			
	Managed care	Total quality	Consolidation	Prevention
Decision support data base for Quality	Consolidates all quality measures Documentation that can be easily transmitted to interested parties	Consolidates all quality measures	Can be used for consolidation and comparison	Supports preparation of educational materials Supports epidemiologic studies
Connect imaging systems		Faster and more accurate Total picture of the patient requires availability of images	Exchange of data across the extended enterprise	
Prototype of electronic medical record	Makes referrals easier	Closes the clinical cycle Faster and more accurate Electronic format helps research and education	Helps to manage the patient across multiple organizations	Total patient profile immediately accessible to all parties with legitimate interest in patient's wellness cycle
Networks in new building	Infrastructure issue—strategy cannot be implemented without it	Infrastructure issue—strategy cannot be implemented without it	Infrastructure issue—strategy cannot be implemented without it	

Appendix—Examples of Technical Architectures

Architecture 1: Stand-alone Computers

The hospital uses "stand-alone" systems. If a hospital had systems from multiple vendors this was the only technical option during the 1960s and 1970s. While increasingly rare, this situtation can still be found. Each system consists of a host and its attached terminals. Each host forms its own "network"—the central processor and its attached terminals and printers. See Figure A.1. This is not a network as the term has come to be understood in the 1980s and 1990s. The terminals are simply display devices, not PCs or workstations. Each host's network is self-contained; it does not provide a connection to any computer outside of itself. A given terminal can only access a single system. Files are synchronized through the periodic exchange of tapes or redundant data entry. A user whose job requires access to two or more systems has to use multiple terminals, and s/he may find that the data bases do not agree, since synchronization, if it does occur, takes place with a lag. Each application looks and feels different. The function keys do different things; the screen layouts are different; the conventions for adding, deleting, and changing data are different.

Obviously, this architecture has the lowest level of access and synchronization, but these shortcomings must be viewed in historical context. This architecture dominated an era when hospital management was concentrating on individual departments, and information technology was in its infancy. There were few capabilities at any network layer, to say nothing of standards. Moreover, U.S. economic conditions were good—they did not require efficient management of resources and customer responsiveness.

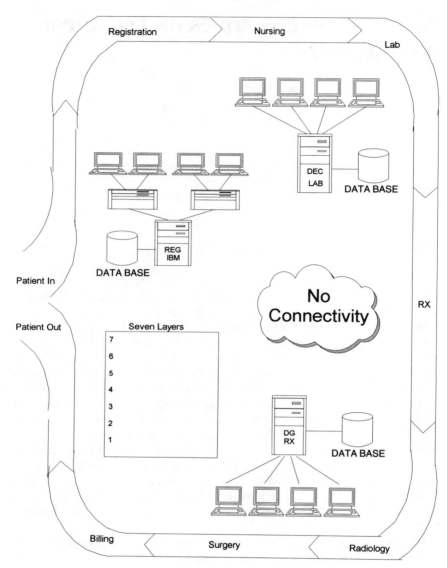

Figure A.1 Stand-alone computers.

Architecture 2: Interfaced Computers

One of the first improvements was to synchronize data bases (at the early stages, they were simply master files). This was done by connecting the hosts over a minimal point-to-point network. See Figure A.2. Typically, this network consisted of point-to-point connections between the CPUs using vendor protocols such as IBM's Bisynch or SDLC. At the same time, each host retained its proprietary network for terminals and other peripherals. If the hosts were in different cities, the X.25 protocol was used for this Wide Area Network. For data base synchronization, one host dials into another host to exchange transactions. Most often, this was

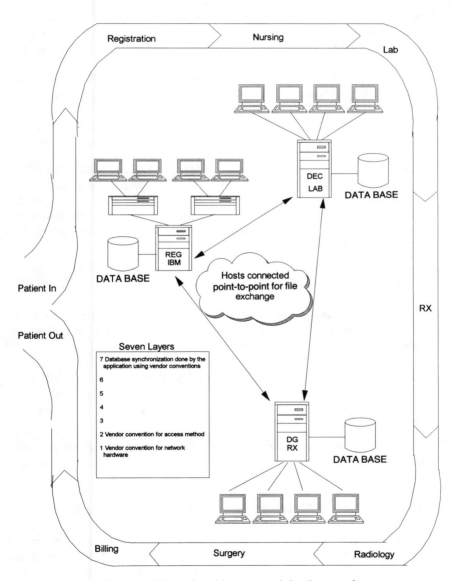

Figure A.2 Interfaced hosts on minimal network.

done in batch mode. These networks were driven by vendor conventions and provided no services above Layer 3. These point-to-point connections among CPUs do not need the routing features provided by Layer 3. The error checking and flow control provided by Layer 4 is done either at Layer 2 or in the application program. Typical applications are minicomputers collecting transaction data during the day and then connecting to an IBM mainframe in the evening to upload these transactions, thereby keeping the centralized consolidated data base synchronized with the local distributed data bases. Each vendor developed his own interfacing conventions, and so there were no standards for synchronizing transactions.

Another method of local connection was to attach the CPUs to a "data switch," which is basically a telephone PBX used for linking computers and their terminals. One computer "dials" into another through the switch. However, throughput was limited. (This switching can also be done through the local phone company. In the latter case, the phone company acts as the network.)

Under this architecture the user is unable to access multiple systems from a single terminal. The user is restricted to using only the applications and data that reside on his/her specific host computer. As a general rule, any activity that requires host-to-host interaction is impossible (such as electronic mail, file transfer, etc.) A Lab technician who desired access to Pharmacy data would need two terminals to perform the job.

Architecture 3: Shared Resources

The next architectural advance was to allow a single terminal to access multiple computers. This is shown in Figure A.3. There are several ways to handle the issue of a single terminal:

1. *Use a "smart" terminal.* It can emulate the characteristics of different vendors' terminals. There is a problem with mapping one keyboard into another. It is also difficult to find a terminal that can handle more than the two or three most common terminal types.

2. *Use a dumb asynchronous terminal.* This is a standard. However, if one has an application that requires features not supported on an asynchronous terminal, the application may not be usable.

There are several different ways to connect to the multiple hosts:

1. *Terminals with multiple lines*: A generic terminal has a separate physical connection for each host that it uses. The user can be connected to two different communications controllers and switch from system to system manually, by throwing a switch. There is a practical problem

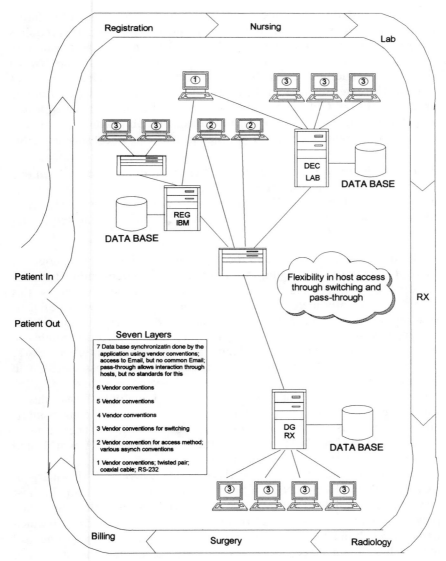

Figure A.3 Terminals access multiple hosts.

with how many hosts can be supported in this fashion. In a dynamic, expanding environment, growth is difficult to accommodate. In Figure A.3, terminals labeled with "1" are connected in this fashion.

2. *Terminals connected through a switch*: The terminal could be connected to a PBX, which does the switching. This switch can also function as a

gateway, translating from one protocol to another. It is difficult to find a terminal that will support the full range of vendor protocols. This requires an asynchronous adapter on the CPU, which functions as a gateway, converting vendor protocols into asynch. Figure A.3 shows a data switch (PBX) in the middle. Terminals that connect to it are labeled with a "2." The switch routes the user to the desired CPU. While the switch could be used for CPU-to-CPU communication as well, it might have difficulty with the throughput. The CPUs, therefore, probably would maintain a direct point-to-point connection, through a vendor protocol such as SDLC or X.25.

3. *Terminals connected through the CPUs*: The terminal is connected to a single host, which has the ability to do "pass-through" and connect the user with another host. This pass-through could be done only when the hosts had the same network protocols. Terminals connected in this fashion are labeled with a "3."

The use of switches started in the 1970s and continued throughout the 1980s. (They are now merging with multiprotocol routers and/or terminal servers.) By giving users the opportunity to access multiple hosts, this architecture greatly increased demand for a variety of network services: printing, remote file access, electronic mail, and so forth across multiple heterogeneous networks. It also greatly increased the need for network management tools. Simple switching provides a rudimentary network; however, it does not provide the higher-level services associated with interoperability. And there is no enterprise-wide network operating system. Even though each user has access to multiple hosts, this is no guarantee of their interoperability for electronic mail, document interchange, data base access, or remote execution of jobs. The de facto standards for terminals are 3270 for the synchronous SNA world, and VT100 for the asynchronous dial-in world.

Around the same time (the early to mid 1970s) TCP/IP emerged. TCP/IP was used with UNIX, a "generic" operating system for the host computers. It provided a way to access multiple hosts with a "generic" network operating system, and bundled many of the services for which demand was building. This networking could be called "heterogeneous" inasmuch as it connected computers from diverse vendors, but it was not heterogeneous in the sense of connecting diverse protocols.

A later variant was to use PCs instead of terminals, since PCs have the capability to emulate the various vendor terminals. A separate network board for each system is installed in the PC, and the PC itself functions as the gateway to the vendor networks. This increases access, but does nothing for synchronization. Moreover, if one has hundreds of users, this is not a very cost-effective strategy, and the management of it is very difficult. The user him/herself functions as the Email "gateway" or the file transfer "gateway." For example, to send a file from the IBM system to the DEC, the user would have to first download it to a PC, and then upload it to the DEC.

Wide Area Networks (WANs) deserve mention. A long-standing issue is how to connect computers in different cities and states without losing speed, accuracy, and functionality. One could also use the switch to dial into a remote computer asynchronously. One could lease a line and multiplex several connections over the same physical wire. Hospitals were less likely than other industries to use a WAN against a large centralized data base. Reservation systems (airlines and hotels) and Automated Teller Machine networks need this capability. There have been some hospital chains that supported multiple hospitals in different cities using a centralized mainframe, and which thus required the use of a WAN. There are two major types of uses: single-purpose transaction processing (reservation systems), where dumb terminals are connected through a series of concentrators and multiplexors; and Email/management systems, where there are multiple hosts connected and which pass messages along. The former case is not a true network, since there is really only a single CPU managing the transactions. In the latter case, many different CPUs are involved. By the end of the 1970s, the two major ways to build WANs were with single vendor solutions (SNA, DECnet, etc.) or with TCP/IP. TCP/IP, however, was more loosely connected (hence the term "Internet"), suited for uses other than "heads-down" transaction processing. The vendor networks, particularly SNA, were well suited for transaction processing.

Architecture 4: Local Area Networks

The next important development, almost a revolution, is the wide installation of PCs and Local Area Networks in the 1980s. Up to this point, networks were primarily oriented toward hosts that controlled terminals, connected point-to-point, and were in hierarchies (the SNA model). This was changed with the introduction of Ethernet, the result of collaboration among DEC, Xerox and Intel. Ethernet is flat and multipoint, in contrast to preceding networks. It allows broadcasts to peers on the same network. All users of this network have a full computer on their desk top. The other LAN products (Token Ring, Arcnet) behaved the same way.

The appearance of LANs is fortuitous in that a new technology has appeared at a time when a new way of doing business is required. This is illustrated in Figure A.4. The competitive position of the United States had changed in the late 1960s and 1970s. Initially, this was not widely realized. It began to be realized in the late 1970s and early 1980s. Hierarchical, command-and-control, mechanistic organizations were going to have to give way to more flexible types of structures, required to adapt

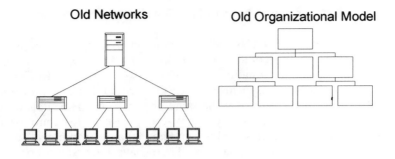

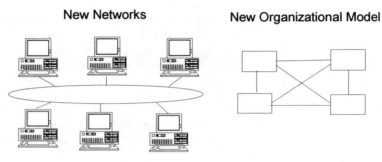

Figure A.4 Alignment of networks and organizations.

to a fast-changing global environment. The hierarchical and point-to-point networks were not really the best model for this new business environment. LANs, with their broadcasting and flattening orientation, more closely resemble the newly emerging business processes. The "lead-lag" effect is shown in Figure A.5. Any business need (e.g., TQM) has technologies and associated methodologies that can support it. The challenge is to make these different learning curves as isochronous as possible; that is, to avoid learning gaps that make it difficult to apply technology effectively.

Ethernet LANs were proposed in the late 1970s, intended for the connection of minicomputers. They were followed in the early 1980s by the introduction of PCs and PC LANs. The early 1980s were marked by a proliferation of vendor conventions for the various network layers. By the mid to late 1980s, the de facto standard for LANs had become Novell. Novell was fine for small work groups, and grew to accommodate whole departments. It was not strong in internetworking, nor were there many standards in place in the mid 1980s. Consequently, there was a considerable amount of variation in the way users got connected to the multiple computers that they needed. In many cases, a user simply installed multiple network interface cards in the PC, and the user functioned as the "human gateway" between the two systems. This is shown in Figure A.6. The user of the Pharmacy Information System, which is the authoritative source of medication-related data, updates a drug record in his system, then "hot-keys" to a session that has been established with the mainframe, and reenters the transaction to keep the two data bases synchronized.

When implemented on a wide scale, this arrangement can lead to considerable management difficulties (rewiring, adding new connections, unique software gateways). This was one of the contributing factors in the development of the concept of a "backbone" network, a common segment of the network over which common traffic flows.

By the end of the 1980s PC LANs became more robust; cabling techniques became standardized; and public telephone networks became more reliable. Some LANs were robust enough to function as enterprise networks; others were more suited for departments and work groups. Ethernet could be used to connect UNIX and DEC hosts. Demand for network functionality exploded, due to the expansion of the functionality on the desk top created by the use of PCs instead of terminals. For the first time, the user has a full computer on the desk top—a full suite of easily accessible applications: word processing, personal data base,

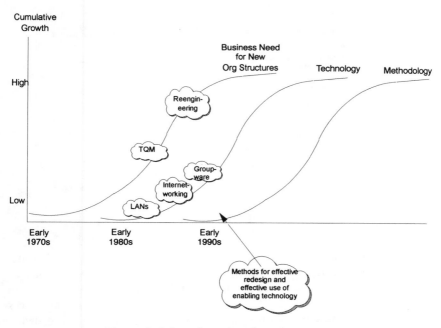

Figure A.5 Lags in various learning curves.

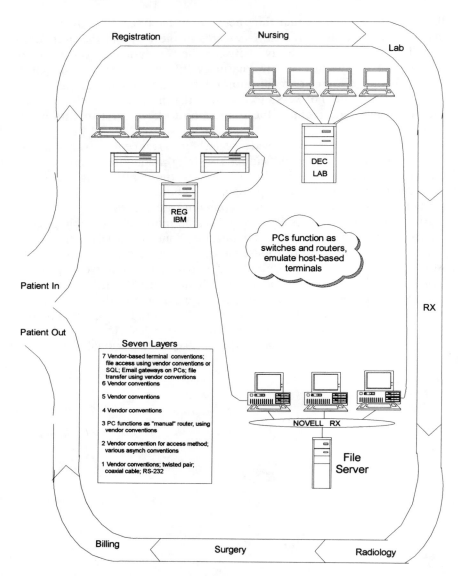

Figure A.6 LANs and PCs.

graphics, spreadsheet, statistics, and other productivity tools. This functionality required the "integrative" functionality of a network such as
Email, file transfer, and database access, and the user gets this locally on
his/her LAN. Many of these LANs lack the ability to link networks
(Layers 3 and 4 designed with single net in mind); however, the growing
use of TCP/IP on minis shows the feasibility of linking networks. Now,

momentum to connect systems across the enterprise starts to grow. Unfortunately, too few users and vendors frame this effort within the context of the seven Layer model.

Recall the three-level model for connectivity used in Figure 6.6: local connection, routing, and end-user functions. Local connection has been achieved; end-user functions have been achieved; the possibility of routing is shown with TCP/IP. It now remains to "glue" all of this together through standards and third-party products. From 1985 to 1993 the industry has been busy providing this. The most important component of this "glue" is the network backbone. This can tie together the user community in a radically new way. It is becoming possible to achieve a close fit between the network and the business processes, and it is now feasible to consider technology to radically restructure the business processes.

Now that there is connectivity, applications must be restructured to take advantage of the capability of communicating with other systems and using their resources. This is forcing vendors to redesign their software, installing APIs that take advantage of the network services.

Architecture 5: Vendor-based Backbone Network

The concept of "internetwork" was originally more oriented toward WANs and host-based systems; the "backbone network" provided a common transmission medium and standard protocols for carrying the internetwork traffic of multiple campus-based LANs, and for attaching a wide variety of PCs and hosts. Some hospitals have used a single vendor's conventions to create a backbone network. Historically, this has meant IBM's SNA. Because of IBM's historical dominance in the computer industry, most vendors had equipment that could provide a gateway to SNA. Figure A.7 shows IBM being used as the network to which non-IBM systems attach. This, however, is a "hierarchical" backbone, since the IBM network is not providing a common medium over which the non-IBM systems can communicate *horizontally* with each other. Rather, it was designed to allow these end systems to communicate *upward* with the IBM host. These gateways were not necessarily two-way, in the sense of peer-to-peer. The network services were all provided by the IBM host. The non-IBM systems did not provide any services to the IBM. IBM's convention is connection-oriented sessions, greatly conditioned by the need to provide a guaranteed level of service to thousands of remote terminals doing transaction processing. This is the opposite of LANs, which are typically connectionless, and creates timing issues among the different networks. This is real internetworking; however, the intermediate systems are all IBM "domains." Routing here is quite different from the routing on a peer-to-peer internet.

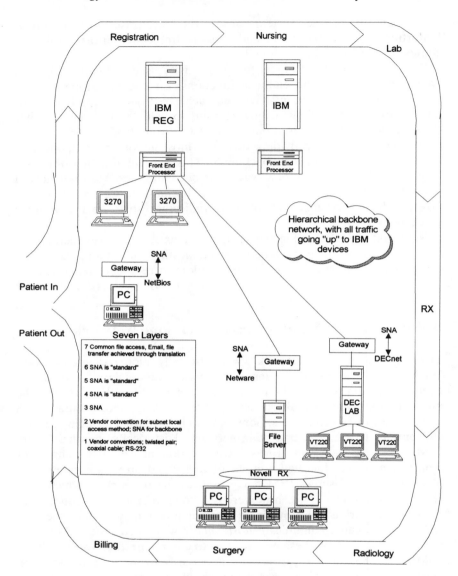

Figure A.7 SNA backbone network.

In Figure A.7 the Novell file server contains a 3270 gateway board in addition to its Arcnet board. This board converts from one type of cabling system to another; it translates from a Novell session to an SNA session; it converts data from EBCDIC to ASCII and viceversa. It might also perform other translations, such as translating from Novell's Email convention to IBM's. The DEC machine has its own gateway board, which performs similar functions. The stand-alone PC's emulation board is its gateway.

In the long run, the custom gateways between vendor conventions and IBM conventions are difficult to manage. They represent the N:N problem that has been discussed previously. Each non-IBM vendor makes changes to his network operating system, mapping its functions to SNA protocols. In theory, a separate gateway could be required for each Layer-7 function: Email, terminal emulation, file transfer, data base access. For every aspect of interoperability, a potential added gateway is required. This gateway does not have to be a separate piece of hardware; it could be just software. For example, the DEC user must have a gateway that converts DEC's protocols for Email into IBM's. Each vendor implements the gateway in a slightly different fashion. Sometimes it is difficult to get the gateway to operate in both directions. Email, file transfer, and data base access might go upward, but not downward.

IBM has developed a protocol named APPN which makes SNA a flatter, peer-oriented transport mechanism, and moves it away from its hierarchical roots. This is a positive thing, for both IBM and the industry. Most large networks within the Fortune 500 companies are SNA nets. Both IBM and the companies themselves will benefit from the use of SNA as a backbone for peer-to-peer connectivity.

For IBM WANs, internetworking is done with X.25. SDLC packets are placed in X.25 packets and routed over the public switched telephone network. Even though X.25 is much faster and more reliable than asynchronous connections over phone lines, its speed and features are not equivalent to that of a LAN, and thus its integrative value is reduced.

With the exception of Digital Equipment Corporation, no other hardware vendor had a sufficiently large installed base or sufficiently rich NOS, enabling it to serve as a proprietary backbone. Although DEC did not start out to provide an open architecture, DECnet was in some ways more conducive to formation of a multivendor backbone network. DecNet was a peer-to-peer network, based on the Ethernet. Over time, DEC has embraced open systems.

Architecture 6: Generic Backbone

Currently, the best way to construct a generic backbone, relatively independent of vendor conventions, is with TCP/IP. During the period 1975–1990, a lot of work was done by universities and government agencies on TCP/IP. TCP/IP literally refers to Layers 4 and 3 of the OSI scheme. TCP (Transmission Control Protocol) performs the functions of the Transport Layer, while IP (Internet Protocol) provides the functions of the Network Layer. In addition, TCP/IP provides functions such as virtual terminal, file transfer, electronic mail, and systems management. One reason why TCP/IP spread so widely is that it was part of the UNIX operating system, which AT&T distributed free to universities. UNIX has been called a "generic operating system," since it can run on a wide variety of hardware platforms. While UNIX is not completely portable, it does provide a generic network system in TCP/IP.

TCP/IP can route messages across a wide variety of subnetworks, using equipment from multiple hardware vendors. For LANs, it most frequently runs over Ethernet (over coaxial cable or twisted pair); for WANs, it can run over X.25 or asynchronous connections. Over time, the higher level features of TCP/IP have been supplemented or replaced by such conventions as NFS (from Sun Microsystems).

Figure A.8 shows the logical configuration for such a backbone. It could have different physical implementations. For example, all terminal devices could be attached to terminal servers; the backbone could consist of a fiber segment, coaxial segments and twisted pair segments. Another variation might be in the gateways. Two of them might be physically housed in the same piece of equipment, which routes and converts multiple protocols and multiple media: for example, twisted pair Ethernet, SNA coaxial, and Token Ring fiber. The same physical device might be used to gateway both the DEC system and the IBM system.

If the hospital continues to use IBM 3270 devices attached to the IBM host, these devices will not be able to display the screens of the Pharmacy and Lab applications. One would need special terminals that can switch from IBM mode to either ANSI or DEC mode.

Many hospitals and medical schools that have a heterogeneous computing environment are moving toward this generic backbone. In cases where the hardware vendor does not provide TCP/IP natively as an extension of the host-based operating system, third parties provide TCP/IP gateways. The hospital can buy the network from a vendor like DEC or HP, but run protocols that are generic (TCP/IP). Routing and protocol processing (translation, tunneling, etc.) require the expenditure of extra computer resources, and can cause bottlenecks.

If a TCP/IP backbone is assumed, then Gateway 1 might be Token Ring to TCP/IP; Gateway 2 would be DECnet to TCP/IP; and Gateway 3 would be Netware to TCP/IP. The details would be accomplished in various ways. The Novell gateway is a second network board in the file server. The PC, for example, does not have a gateway; it is attached directly to the backbone and it is already running the TCP/IP software. These gateways work in various ways. Some perform "translation," whereby the network protocols are translated into TCP/IP, sent over the network, and then translated to the target network operating system. Another technique is "tunneling," whereby the full Netware packet is encapsulated within a TCP/IP packet. When it reaches its destination, the shell is stripped away.

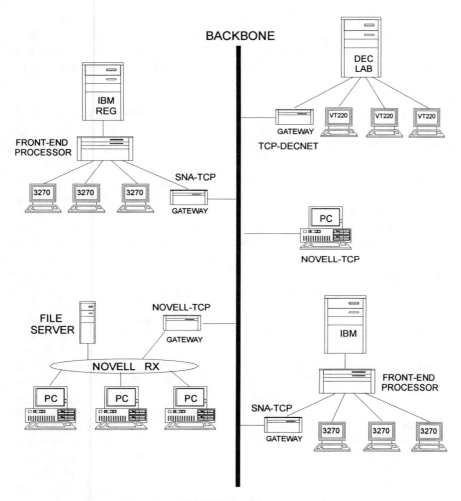

Figure A.8 TCP/IP backbone network.

While conceptually simple, current backbone networks are very complex because this logical unity is achieved by assembling an array of
intermediate devices that perform protocol translation rather than
standards-based protocol layering. These components, and the end user
systems, were not designed to a single standard. The components, using
their own proprietary conventions, translate from one vendor convention
to another. This translation and conversion concern features at all 7
layers: naming conventions, addressing schemes, routing schemes, email
formats, file transfer schemes, data base access schemes, as well as timing
and sequencing schemes. The complexity behind Figure A.8 can be seen

in the scenario of a pharmacist wanting to check diagnosis, medications, and outcomes data for a patient's previous visits. The pharmacist is located on the pharmacy network, while the patient data is contained on the IBM system for registration. The following things have to happen:

1. The pharmacist initiates a second network session, on the IBM registration host. SNA terminal emulation software is loaded on the PC, and software on the Novell network builds a packet containing a request for an SNA session on the IBM machine.

2. The hospital is using a TCP/IP backbone. Novell can provide a gateway to an SNA network, and it can also serve as a gateway to a TCP/IP network. However, can it also "tunnel" the SNA session request in a TCP/IP envelope, or must the gateway be direct to SNA? This gateway must support a connectionless session on the Novell side, but a connection-oriented session on the IBM side.

3. If it is possible to perform this tunneling, what will be lost in the translation from Novell to TCP/IP and then from TCP/IP to SNA?

4. The pharmacist has an array of end-user PC productivity tools, such as email, data base query, and file exchange. Even if he can reach the IBM system, can his tools work with the tools on the IBM side? It is one thing to have parallel network sessions using terminal emulation, which is the simplest of connectivity scenarios. It is quite another thing to achieve interoperability of end-user productivity tools.

It should be noted that the user is *not* accessing another system directly from within his primary application. Rather, he suspends the primary application and accesses a second application on another machine. When he is finished with the second application, he terminates it and returns to the first (suspended) application. The Pharmacy application will not automatically access the HIS to find out the allergy information. Developments in Microsoft Windows like OLE (object linking and embedding) will have a major impact on the ability of an application to call another remote application transparently to the user.

Bibliography

Blois, Marsden S. *Information and Medicine: The Nature of Medical Descriptions*. Berkeley and Los Angeles: University of California Press, 1984.

Bruce, Thomas A. *Designing Quality Databases with IDEF1X Information Models*. New York: Dorset House Publishing, 1992.

Cash, James I., F. Warren McFarlan, James L. McKenney, and Michael R. Vitale. *Corporate Information Systems Management: Text and Cases*. 3rd ed. Homewood, Illinois: Richard D. Irwin, 1992.

DeLuca, Joseph M. with Owen Doyle. *Health Care Information Systems: An Executive's Guide for Successful Management*. Chicago, Illinois: American Hospital Publishing, 1991.

Digital Equipment Corporation. *H.I.S. Management Guide*. Digital Equipment Corporation, 1988. Also by Digital Equipment Corporation: *Open Systems Handbook: A Guide to Building Open Systems*. Maynard, MA: 1991.

Dorenfest, Sheldon. *Hospital Information Systems: State of The Art*. Northbrook, Illinois: Sheldon I. Dorenfest & Associates, 1988.

Goldberg, Alan J. and Robert A. Buttaro. *Hospital Departmental Profiles*. 3rd ed. Chicago, IL: American Hospital Publishing, 1990.

Hammer, Michael and James Champy. *Reengineering the Corporation: A Manifesto for Business Revolution*. New York: Harper Business, 1993.

Hancock, Bill. *Designing and Implementing Ethernet Networks*. 2nd ed. Wellesley, MA: QED Information Sciences, Inc., 1988.

Harrington, John J., Timothy J.R. Benson, and Andrew L. Spector "IEEE P1157 Medical Data Interchange (MEDIX) Committee Overview and Status Report," *Proceedings of the Fourteenth Annual Symposium on Computer Applications in Medical Care* (IEEE Computer Society Press, 1990), pp. 230–234.

HL-7 Working Group. *Health Industry Level 7 Interface Standards, Version 2.1.* 1990.

Institute of Electrical and Electronics Engineers. *P1073 Overview & Architecture* [Unapproved Draft]. Piscataway, NJ: IEEE, 1991.

Institute of Electrical and Electronics Engineers. *P1157 Medical Data Interchange Overview* [Unapproved Draft]. Piscataway, NJ: IEEE, 1990.

Lindberg, Donald A.B. and Betsy L. Humphreys. "The UMLS Knowledge Sources: Tools for Building Better User Interfaces," *Proceedings of the Fourteenth Annual Symposium on Computer Application in Medical Care* (IEEE Computer Society Press, 1990), pp. 121–125.

Loomis, Mary E.S. *The Database Book.* New York: Macmillan, 1987.

MacKinnon, Dennis, William McCrum, and Donald Sheppard. *An Introduction to Open Systems Interconnection.* New York: W.H. Freeman, 1990.

Malamud, Carl. *Analyzing DECnet/OSI Phase V.* New York: Van Nostrand Reinhold, 1991.

Martin, James. *Information Engineering.* 3 vols. Englewood Cliffs, NJ: Prentice Hall, 1990.

Nolan, Lorene S. and Michael M. Shabot. "The P1073 Medical Information Bus Standard: Overview and Benefits for Clinical Users," *Proceedings of the Fourteenth Annual Symposium on Computer Applications in Medical Care* (IEEE Computer Society Press, 1990), pp. 216–219.

Omachonu, Vincent K. *Total Quality and Productivity Management in Health Care Organizations.* Norcross, GA: Institute of Industrial Engineers, 1991.

Porter, Michael E. *Competitive Advantage.* New York: Free Press, 1985.

Porter, Michael E. and Victor E. Millar. "How Information Gives You Competitive Advantage," *Harvard Business Review*, July–August 1985.

Ranade, Jay and George C. Sackett. *Introduction to SNA Networking.* New York: McGraw-Hill, 1989.

Sneider, Richard. *Management Guide to Health Care Information Systems.* Rockville, MD: Aspen Publishers, 1987.

Starr, Paul. *The Social Transformation of American Medicine.* New York: Basic Books, 1982.

Glossary

APPN: *Advanced Peer-to-Peer Networking*. An IBM protocol allowing SNA networks to communicate in a peer-to-peer fashion with non-IBM systems that use other routing protocols.

API: *Application Programming Interface*. The specification for how an application program calls an operating system program or function.

Bridge: A device used to connect two networks that have the same Data Link Protocol (OSI Layer 2), but which have different physical media, e.g., coaxial cable versus microwave (OSI Layer 1).

Candidate Entity: A business object discovered during the early phases of building a data model and subjected to further analysis in order to determine whether it should be included in the data model.

Cardinality: A statement about the number of entities that must appear at either end of a relationship, usually expressed as 1-to-many, one-to-0/1/many, etc.

CRC: *Commitment, Concurrency, and Recovery*. An OSI protocol for verifying that resources are available on other network nodes to perform a given operation and for checking that the operation was indeed performed. It is useful in distributed data bases, where multiple systems have to store the same record at the same time.

CFO: *Chief Financial Officer*.

CIO: *Chief Information Officer*.

CLNS: *Connectionless Network Service*. An OSI Protocol at the Session Layer (Layer 5), allowing two applications to communicate without maintaining the overhead of a connection.

CONS: *Connection-Oriented Network Service*. An OSI Protocol at the Session Layer (Layer 5), allowing two applications to communicate over a connection.

Conceptual Schema: The representation of data in a form that is independent of its physical storage or its external appearance (presentation format).

DBMS: *Data Base Management System*. A program that manages the storage and access of data independently of the programs that use this data.

DCE: *Distributed Computing Environment*. A suite of connectivity protocols developed by the Open Software Foundation (OSF).

DEC: *Digital Equipment Corporation*.

DNA: *Digital Network Architecture*. The technical framework of DEC's network architecture.

DRG: *Diagnosis Related Group*. A system for classifying and grouping health care diagnosis, for purposes of reimbursement and statistical analysis.

EDI: *Electronic Data Interchange*. The practice of exchanging business transactions electronically (e.g., electronic purchase orders, electronic invoices, etc.). It also refers to the standards which specify the structure of these electronic transactions.

Entity: A person, place, thing, or event about which data is kept. Each intance of an entity must be uniquely distinguishable.

Existence Dependence: In data modeling, the case that one entity can not be created until another entity has already been created. For example, a Purchase Order entity is existence-dependent on a Customer entity.

Gateway: Loosely defined, a device used to connect two different networks, such as IBM's SNA and DEC's DECnet. In this case, the gateway would provide conversion and/or translation not just at Layers 2 and 3, but also at Layer 4 and above, since there are session, data format, and interprocess communication differences.

GOSIP: *Government OSI Protocols*. A United States government specified subset of the international OSI standards.

Institutional Account: A type of account in hospitals, particularly tertiary-care hospitals, used to collect charges for ambulatory services performed for other hospitals.

IS: *Information System*.

ISO: *International Standards Organization*. An international standards-promulgating agency, responsible for the OSI standards.

ISP: *International Standards Profile*. An internationally agreed upon set of OSI protocols, at several or all layers of the OSI model, which provide a total "solution" to a business problem. For example, MAP defines the protocols needed at all seven layers for automating the manufacturing process.

IT: *Information Technology*.

JCAHO: *Joint Commission on Accreditation of Healthcare Organizations*.

Knowledge Base: A special type of data base that contains a representation of the knowledge possessed by a human expert in a particular area of endeavor.

Legacy System: A popular term that refers to the older information systems within an organization. Legacy systems are typically developed with software tools that do not allow connectivity, with stand-alone designs, or on obsolete hardware. The dilemma caused by legacy systems is that they constrain systems development because they collect most of the data that feeds the more modern systems. Moreover, their obsolete technology prevents the understanding of them that is needed to replace them.

MAP: *Manufacturing Automation Protocol.* An International Standards Profile, or suite of OSI protocols, for the automation of manufacturing on the shop floor. Its strongest proponents have been General Motors and Boeing.

MIB: *Medical Information Bus.* An International Standards Profile, or suite of OSI protocols, for the exchange of data among bedside devices, including data for their control.

Non-key Attribute: An attribute of and entity that does not serve to identify it.

OLE: *Object Linking and Embedding.* A Microsoft Corporation convention for the exchange of data and functionality among Windows applications. It has become a de-facto standard.

OSI: *Open Systems Interconnection.* The ISO's standards for inter-operability across heterogeneous networks. The 7-layer reference model is just a part of OSI.

OSI Stack: A set of programs that provide the network services specified by OSI in the manner specified by OSI. The programs are "stacked," whereby a given service provides a certain amount of functionality at its layer and then calls upon a lower-layer service for additional functionality. There are strict rules governing how these services may call each other.

PDU: *Protocol Data Unit.* The control data that each network layer adds to the packet. The original user data (e.g., an Email message) is thus surrounded by successive layers of protocol data, which is used by the respective network layer on the receiving end.

Primary Key: The attribute or attributes that serve to identify each instance of an entity.

RDBMS: *Relational Data Base Management System.* A data base management system that behaves according to the relational model of data, in which data is represented as tables, records are stored as rows of the tables, and data elements are stored as columns within the rows.

RFP: *Request for Proposal.*

Router: A device connecting network segments for different networks. It functions at layer 3 of the ISO model and determines the best path for routing the message.

SAA: *Systems Application Architecture.* An IBM architecture for developing applications that can run across multiple hardware platforms and operating systems, but which look the same to the end user and have the same API for programmers.

SNA: *System Network Architecture.* IBM's architecture for computer networking.

SQL: *Structured Query Language.* An international standard language for defining and manipulating the data in relational data bases. Some non-relational data bases also have SQL as their "front-end."

TCP/IP: *Transmission Control Protocol/Internet Protocol.* Not an official OSI standard, but a non-proprietary, defacto standard for connecting networks at layers 4 and 3, respectively. It originated in Unix networks, but has become the standard for heterogeneous networks as well.

TOP: *Technical Office Protocol.* An International Standards Profile, or suite of OSI protocols, for the automation of administrative functions within a manufacturing environment. Its strongest proponents have been General Motors and Boeing.

TQM: *Total Quality Management.*

VSAM: *Virtual Storage Access Method.* An IBM convention for the organization, storage, and access of disk-based files. VSAM provides these services to application programs.

Index